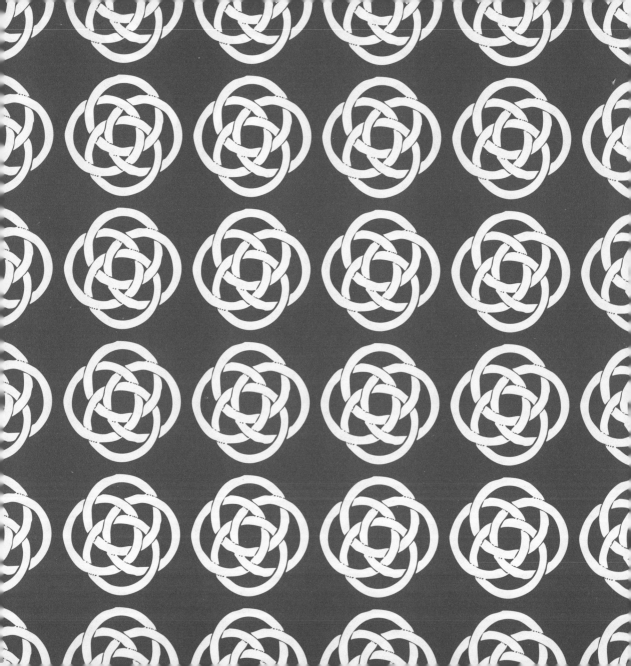

Dedication

To my husband, Len LaBrae, the samurai in my bedroom

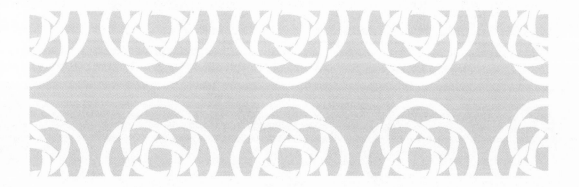

CONTENTS

INTRODUCTION

The art of seduction begins in the discovery of what is sensual all around you. The graceful movement of the female form; the whisper of a witty phrase; the eye-appealing color, texture, and placement of food; tasteful décor; a sense of ritual and ceremony, even an atmosphere of playfulness—these not only please your senses, but also engage your emotions. They elevate your enjoyment of sex beyond a monotone state of organic activity into a noble and pleasurable pursuit.

Seduction is an art that tantalizes, titillates, and touches your soul as well as your body. It can enhance your life in the modern world, where the intrusion of fast-paced technology and stress can interfere with sex, often dehumanizing it.

The idea of coupling the physical act of lovemaking with spirituality, formal traditions, and play led me to a place that has long fascinated me: Japan. Japan, in turn, led me to write this book.

Pleasure in Japan is about creating something exquisite and wonderful that transcends the mundane, humdrum activities of life. The Japanese believe the pleasure of sex at its best is a total package: It involves bathing, cuisine, song and dance, good company, and finally, lovemaking. Every detail is regulated by honored customs, superstitions, cultural refinements, witty repartee, and artistic ceremonies that have taken shape over the centuries. The hint of the hidden, the mysterious, and even the clandestine has only made it more enticing. There is nothing crude or coarse about this ideal, and yet it is so persuasive that even the modern sex trade in some ways turns to it for inspiration.

I am no stranger to Japan, having spent many years working for Japanese companies. However, learning the art of kimono with a *sensei*, teacher, whose family had been in that business for more than four hundred years, led me to explore the sensuous roots of Japanese women by studying literature and art. There I discovered the essence of their seduction techniques. I found it not in observing what was on the surface, but as in so many things Japanese, in peeling off the outer layer and looking inside. This has intrigued me for years and kept me coming back to Japan, studying the culture, traditions, and rituals of seduction.

In my explorations, I have encountered many fascinating women: Early empresses possessed legendary powers of enchantment and in some instances were warriors. Ladies of the Heian period (794–1192) established ideals of beauty and were accomplished poets and masters of innuendo, intrigue, and romance in the imperial court. Courtesans of the Edo period (1615–1868) were the classic women of pleasure, trendsetters who made an art of sexual technique and the refined arts of song, dance, music, and conversation—talents later epitomized by the geisha. The last of the geisha still carry on this elegant and sensual tradition. Even modern bar hostesses and soapland girls look to the ideals of the past to give a small gloss of beauty and refinement to otherwise tawdry professions. All these women have one thing in common—*itoke*, sex appeal—and they all contribute to my book in different and evocative ways.

I discovered that in earlier times the Japanese were fond of instructing on sexual methods by means of pictorial hanging scrolls whose graphic depictions were also exquisite works of art. Men learned about sex from books "like you learn rules for making a garden."[1] Yet, seeking information on the art of seduction, I encountered no *meishoki*, guidebooks, on how to seduce a lover. I knew then I would have to find my own way by exploring the

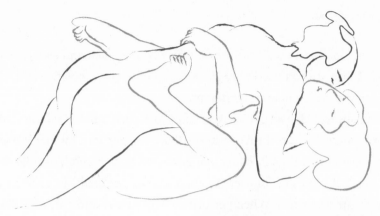

A couple making love in Old Edo,
from a woodblock print

lives and habits of sensual Japanese women throughout the centuries. And, I knew that while these sexy, beautiful court ladies, courtesans, and geisha could offer models for learning the pleasure of seduction, we live in a different place and time. I would need a book for the tastes of the empowered Western woman of today: you.

I gathered together Japanese customs and traditions, blended them with erotic and sensual ways of our own, and assembled it all into a step-by-step guide that can help *you* perfect the art of seduction so you and your lover can experience better sex on different levels, where the taste of love is sweeter, the pace more relaxed, and the love play more succulent. In this book, you will explore how you can benefit from the sensual secrets of the fascinating women of Japan by using your erotic senses of sight, hearing, smell, touch, and taste to prepare your mind, body, and soul to experience the ultimate pleasure of good sex. With Japanese poems, stories, history, and art for inspiration, you will learn how to seduce: to enhance the beauty of your body and your spirit, to flirt with gesture, dress, conversation, and wit, and to tempt with music, atmosphere, bathing, food, movement, and in so many other subtle ways. Finally, you will end your journey with explicit and evocative lessons in the art of making love. All you need to begin is sexual curiosity, a positive attitude, and an open mind to try something new and different.

I have always believed good sex satisfies *both* partners beyond the ultimate physical release. Seduction is like the elusive butterfly that captures your fascination with her colorful wings always in motion, dazzling maneuvers forever graceful, sinfully evocative, and *never* boring. It is a journey for every woman who understands the exciting and sensual component of the mating ritual. When performed with finesse and a clear understanding of how you can give as well as receive pleasure, seduction can be a rewarding and exciting experience at any age.

I would like to acknowledge the tireless efforts of Kay Segal, who helped me shape this book, always keeping my vision in mind; also, the artwork of Yelena Zhavoronkova for giving life and movement to my words; and mostly Peter Goodman, my publisher, whose faith and belief in me and in this book from the very beginning never wavered. *Domo arigato gozaimashita.*

J.B.

THE JAPANESE ART OF SEX

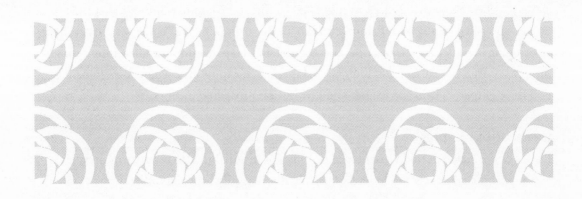

JAPANESE WOMEN THROUGHOUT THE AGES

EMPRESSES

Seven empresses ruled ancient Japan. Most fascinating was the mysterious, semi-legendary Himiko, credited with unifying the country in the third century A.D. and making contact with China. A shaman who lived in seclusion, by day she was attended by women; by night male slaves gratified her sexual desires, as suggested by director Masahiro Shinoda in a 1974 film.[1] Suiko, who ruled jointly with Prince Shotoku Taishi[2] from A.D. 592 to 628, was instrumental in bringing literary arts, a legal code, and Buddhism to Japan, and promoted international diplomacy. In A.D. 710, Genmei built Nara, Japan's first capital city, where four empresses and three emperors held the scepter and civilization prospered until 782.[3]

HEIAN COURT LADIES

Ladies of the Heian period were judged not just for beauty but also for taste in dress and accomplishments in arts and letters, especially the elegantly brushed calligraphy in which they wrote their renowned poetry. Under their embroidered Chinese jackets, they adorned themselves in multiple robes of exquisite silk, arranged so the up to forty successive layers of beautifully matched colors could be seen and admired at the neck and sleeves.[4] With long,

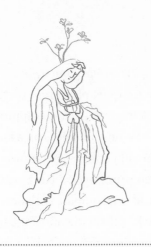

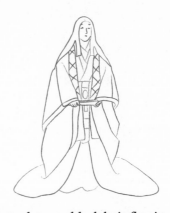

A goddess and a Heian court lady
wearing a many-layered kimono

Rapunzel-esque black hair flowing down their backs often reaching the floor, they were among the most sensual women in Japanese history. As Sarashina Nikki wrote in her diary in 1037, "I was dressed in an eight-fold *uchigi* (outer robe) of deep and pale chrysanthemum colors, and over it I wore the outer flowing robe of deep red silk."[5]

Two women who exemplified this ideal were the literary geniuses Murasaki Shikibu (978–1015) and Sei Shonagon (ca. 966–1025). In mirroring the aesthetic preoccupations that permeated every part of court life, from manner of dress to way of living, to its unique perspective on the art of seduction, their works also laid down the classic templates for exquisite and elegant taste. Murasaki Shikibu wrote the most famous work in Japanese literature, considered the first novel ever written, *Genji Monogatari*, "The Tale of Genji." Sei Shonagon wrote *Makura no Soshi*, "The Pillow Book," an erotic journal of memories and fantasies that captured the spirit of the time, including the popular "phallus game,"[6] which measured the prowess of a man and his ability to keep an erection.

However, it wasn't all sex and games. Heian ladies also understood how to savor

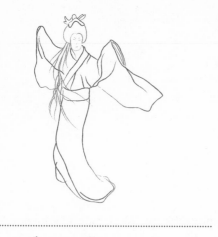

*A courtesan dancing, wearing a
kimono with winged sleeves*

life according to *miyabi*, courtly beauty,[7] best described as the quiet pleasures experienced by smelling a fragrant perfume, appreciating the delicate blending of colors on a kimono, or feeling the silky softness of a flower petal between your fingers.[8] Nothing in the Western world can compare with how aesthetics played a role in the life of the senses. In that manner, *miyabi* could also refer to the art of seduction, whether a woman attracted a man by the elegant movement of her long sleeves or by her skillful playing of the lute. It is this sense of *miyabi* that Heian ladies handed down to successive generations of sensual Japanese women, especially the fascinating courtesan.

COURTESANS

Courtesans, part of Japanese society from ancient times, operated actively into the twentieth century. Originally called *saburuko*, "ones who serve,"[9] their titles changed over the eras. They occupied a hierarchy according to the cost of their services, from the lowest ranking *hashi*, ordinary prostitute, to the elegant, refined *tayu* of the *karyukai*, "world of flowers and willows," as this life was called. Most famously romantic were the *tayu* of Edo's licensed district, the Yoshiwara. These women with their seductive wiles were the leaders of fashion, copied by women of all classes as explained by Ejima Kiseki (1667–1736) in *Characters of Worldly Young Women* (1717): "mother and daughter . . . ape the manners of harlots and

Ukiyo, "Floating World"

Ukiyo means "floating world," originally a Buddhist term used in the Heian period to describe the sadness and impermanence of life. During the Edo period, when *bons vivants* of the time sought a word to express their foray into the erotic and seductive world of the senses,[a] *ukiyo* acquired a new, trendier meaning by making a pun of the word *uki*. Meaning both "sorrowful" and "floating," it came to refer to the transient pleasures of the gay quarters. The word also came to be associated with a certain chic, a savoir-faire in the arts. This included life in the brothels, which had its own set of rules and guides governing the behavior expected of its patrons and denizens.[b]

A remarkable period of distinctive, highly creative artistic traditions and sexual exploration arose from this fertile environment: the Genroku era (1688–1703), where sex and money ruled.[c] Sexual pleasure in all forms was an end unto itself, in any and every persuasion, including autoerotica, bisexuality, and homosexuality. In the Yoshiwara, the famous brothel district of Edo (now Tokyo), writers composed lyrical poems and artists made sketches for graphically illustrated "pillow books." Sex, art, and literature culminated in erotic and exquisite pictures known as *shunga*, "spring drawings," which featured prominent displays of both male and female genitalia, and explicit references in satirical masterpieces like Ihara Saikaku's *Koshoku Gonin Onna*, "Five Women Who Loved Love" (1686).

courtesans."[10] Prostitution was a widely accepted and very active aspect of society, but certain things set *tayu* apart as women of the senses, such as their intricate hairstyles and extravagant kimonos tied in front instead of the more traditional back.

Customers were very particular about picking out a girl and often consulted *Shikido Okagami*, "The Great Mirror of the Way of Love," by Hatakeyama Kizan, as well as *Hidensho*, "Secret Teachings," by Okumura Sanshiro, that listed both a girl's physical attributes and her cultural achievements. But, the highest-ranking *tayu* could turn down a client if she found him distasteful.

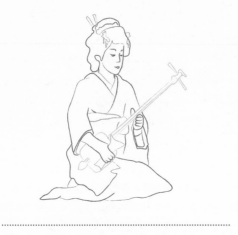

A geisha playing the shamisen,
a three-stringed lute

GEISHA

Around this time, a mysterious and desirable creature surfaced in this fascinating world of seduction: The geisha, considered the most artistic and accomplished woman in the history of Japan. The term is best understood by the meanings of the two ideograms used to write the word: *gei*, "art," and *sha*, "person." In the seventeenth century, "geisha" referred to any person engaged in a profession of artistic accomplishment.[11] Male geisha, who entertained the guests of the courtesans with ribald jokes and antics, were referred to as *hokan*, jesters.[12] Young female entertainers called *odoriko*, literally meaning "dancing child," began by likening themselves after male geisha. Performing for high-ranking courtesans,[13] they evolved into elegant, stylized ideals of femininity. The geisha was strictly forbidden to compete with the courtesan, but when the days of the Yoshiwara and high courtesans came to an end, the geisha emerged as the premier provider of elegant entertainment in the "world of flowers and willows."

Geisha apprentices, with their long, long sleeves and even longer hanging sashes, spent their childhood years learning literary and artistic skills, as well as beauty skills—from her graceful silhouette to her soft voice to her slightest gesture—that enhanced her mystique and her power over men. Whether dancing or playing an instrument like the *shamisen* (lute), each girl was expected to excel in her chosen art, as well as in *chanoyu* (tea ceremony) and *kado* or *ikebana* (flower arranging). She was also expected to be a witty conversationalist. The geisha was known and respected for her loyalty and her emotional commitment and for her skills and artistic accomplishments.

Geisha flourished in a golden period that lasted from the 1860s up to the beginning of the twentieth century, but a few still carry on this elegant tradition. In them, what began as the ancient idea of *miyabi*, and evolved into the aesthetic of the courtesan, became a more modern kind of artfulness and sensuality.

HOSTESSES, SOAPLAND GIRLS, AND THE TAKARAZUKA ALL-GIRL REVUE

The days of opulence, grand castles, and sumptuous brothels are gone. But, according to a recent study, ten percent of men in Japan pay for sex at least once a month.[14] Women today in the *mizushobai*, "water trade" or sex business, ply their wares in other ways.

By the 1920s, *jokyu*, "cafe girls," began to rival geisha. They are considered the predecessors of the present day *hosutesu*, "bar hostesses." Some bars are small intimate places, the waiting rooms from the old prostitution houses; others are sleek, modern establishments with live, usually nude or semi-nude, entertainment. Hostesses are expected to engage in a fantasy world, pampering the customer and allowing him to believe he could be the man in her life. They also go on what are called *dohan*, "couples

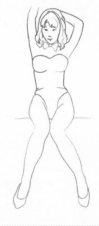

A modern soapland girl, waiting for a customer

dates," to a restaurant with their customers, then bring them back to the club for a nightcap. Young women also engage in a practice known as *enjo kosai*, "compensated dating." This is a "sugar daddy" system where older men go out with younger girls. Japanese culture does not make it acceptable for the girl to accept cash for the relationship, so the men give the girls gifts. Soapland girls, like the *yuna*, "bath maidens," of old, provide services, sexual and otherwise, for a fee in bathhouses. A different kind of seduction also goes on under the footlights, including strip clubs and the male-impersonating Takarazuka All-Girl Revue (made famous by the 1957 film *Sayonara* based on the novel by James Michener), while soft-porn cinema actresses seduce men from the privacy of their own bedrooms through television monitors.

Chapter 1

KOKONO-TOKORO:
"THE NINE POINTS OF BEAUTY"

Our world is different from the ordinary world. If we were to dress ourselves like ordinary girls, how on earth would we manage to attract lovers?

Naoe, courtesan from the Shinmachi pleasure quarters of Osaka (1789)[1]

In Japan, sensuous women throughout history have refined the art of beauty to a simple and easy-to-follow guide known as *kokono-tokoro*, the "Nine Points of Beauty": eyes, mouth, head, hands, feet, spirit, standing posture, seductive air, and voice.[2] Among these, perhaps "spirit" was the hardest to put your finger on. A courtesan who did it all to perfection had a special quality or spirit called *hari*. A woman with *hari* was dazzlingly sharp, gorgeous no matter what her features, smoldering with élan, and irresistible even with her clothes *on*.[3]

Erotica was hardly taboo in Edo Japan, but instead of the female nude, the emphasis was on portraying a woman's physical beauty by showing her poise, the proportions of the contours and features of her face, her hair coifed in the latest fashion, and the elegant grace with which she wore her magnificent kimono.[4] In *ukiyoe*, woodblock prints from this era, clothed women radiate an erotically stimulating sensuality. Looking at these images of beautiful women was often referred to as "reading with one hand."[5] These women all followed the Nine Points of Beauty, and all had *hari.*

What makes them so relevant to the art of seduction is that Japan is a society where sexual activity is celebrated as a part of life, and seduction has to be sophisticated as well as innovative in order to arouse and stimulate the male libido. What better way to excite a man than by adapting these Nine Points of Beauty into your daily regimen and perfecting your own kind of *hari*? With five points for physical beauty and four for beauty of character, this is a rich and fulfilling regimen that will make you feel dramatic and sexy on the outside, and your inner beauty will shine through in self-confidence as you embark on your next seductive adventure in the bedroom.

EYES

> But it was above all her eyes which attracted attention—sparkling with intelligence beneath arched and particularly well-marked eyebrows.[6]
>
> Referring to O-Koi, a famous
> nineteenth-century Shinbashi geisha

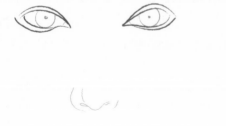

The dramatically lined eyes of the
geisha attract attention

The makeup of the geisha was dramatic. Nothing was used on the eyelashes; the preference instead was to create depth with eyeliner. A young *maiko*, apprentice geisha, drew the area around her eyes and eyebrows in red and black; as she matured into a geisha,[7] she used more black to add depth to the physical

Geisha Makeup

With its potpourri of little pots and brushes and bright colors, Geisha makeup fascinated Westerners.[a] The white that completely covered her face, called *oshiroi*,[b] could be traced back to the Heian period, when Japan was greatly influenced by the court of China, where the custom originated. Cruse, as it was called, gave a flat, almost mask-like quality.[c] Ironically, it was lead-based, which aged skin prematurely and sometimes caused death.[d] The white makeup used later was gentle and safe. Geisha wore it on their hands and arms below the elbow, as well as on their faces. After the painting was finished, powder was rubbed gently on the skin with a puff.[e]

Traditional geisha makeup was daring as well as symbolic, especially at the nape of the neck. Using a template, two serpent-like lines were left unpainted, three lines[f] for special ceremonies. These created erotic "tongues" of bare flesh, hinting at a woman's genitalia.[g]

appearance of her eyes as well as to convey a deepening spirituality within her professional status. Eyebrows, *mayu,* were a distinctive element. The face was given a natural "lift" by tweezing the entire eyebrow and then painting in a higher one. The shape was so important that if she didn't pencil them in properly, she had to remove *all* her makeup and begin again. The perfect eyebrow in the Edo period was *katsura no mayu* ". . . delicately shaped like a new moon."[8] *Katsura* means the redbud or Judas tree, which, according to Chinese legend, grew on the moon and referred to the crescent moon shape of the brow. "And if I said, ' . . . my eyebrows are itching . . . ' it meant my lover would be visiting me soon."[9]

Eye Tips

- Geisha kept their eyes lowered when they entered a room, revealing a sweep of pink-red or black eyeliner on their upper and lower eyelids. Be mindful that eye shadow can cake in the crease of your eyelids if you apply it too thickly. First, brush your eyelids with a light translucent powder, then apply your eye shadow

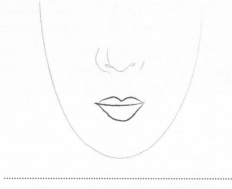

to help prevent caking in the creases. Careful blending of the colors on your lids is the secret to creating dramatic but tasteful eye makeup.

• Long before the geisha, the ladies of the Heian period, who lived most of their lives hidden indoors, created an air of mystery when they peeked at their lovers from behind latticed shades and woven screens. Wearing sunglasses is a modern way to be dramatic and mysterious.

MOUTH

The lips have been idealized throughout Japanese history. Erotic novelist Ihara Saikaku (1642–93) wrote, "... her lovely lips looked like the topmost leaves of Takao in full autumnal glory."[10] Geisha used safflower lipstick to color their lips an intense peony red, giving the mouth the appearance of a flower petal.[11] Crystallized sugar melted into the lipstick created a succulent luster. In the past, a tiny puckered mouth, *ochoboguchi*, was considered the most desirable, which is why *maiko* colored only the lower lip.[12]

GEISHA SKIN CARE

Her complexion had the delicate tint of a single-petalled cherry blossom.[13]

How did geisha and courtesans have such beautiful skin? During the Heian period, court ladies like Lady Murasaki washed their faces with a silk washing bag filled with a combination of rice bran or *azuki* bean powders and camellia nuts. This face wash cleans the skin thoroughly without stripping your complexion of its natural oils[14] because rice bran, *nuka*, contains B-complex vitamins and vitamin E.[15] Geisha traditionally used nightingale droppings to cleanse the face. This pale yellow face cream is famous for giving the skin a pearl-like pallor. With special care taken to remove the odor it is still sold today in small packets, but is very expensive.

SKIN CARE AND MAKEUP TIPS

- You can make your own *nuka*, rice bran wash, at home: Fill a small silk drawstring bag with finely powdered rice bran (use *only* pure rice bran, found at natural health food stores). Soak the bag for a few minutes in a hot bath, then squeeze. When the milky liquid seeps through, the rice bran wash is ready to use. Wash your face with the silk bag in a gently massaging motion. The soft fabric performs a gentle sloughing of your face while the cleansing ingredients within nourish, polish, and purify your complexion.[16] You can use the silk bag two or three times (hang it up in a dry place), then refill with fresh rice bran powder.

- Geisha teahouses were designed to make the most of natural light. Do as the geisha did and apply your makeup in a natural light. You'll know much better what the colors look like against your complexion.

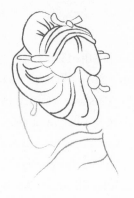

....

A traditional coiffure, like this one from the
Edo period, could be formal and dramatic

HEAD

Lady Murasaki in the Heian period wrote, "Her [Lady Dainagon] hair is three inches longer than her height."[17] As so many depictions in art make clear, for centuries Japanese women wore their hair as long as possible: the more luxuriant the hair, the more evocative its suggestion of sensuality.[18] In Edo times, women used so much water to wash their hair that public baths charged them higher rates. In those days, hair was washed only once a month, but was meticulously groomed daily with a fine-toothed comb and perfumed oils.[19]

Likewise appreciating the seductiveness of long tresses, geisha took a different approach. Their elaborate coifs were designed for dramatic yet traditional formality, and also were symbolic. You could tell whether or not a geisha was a virgin by the way she wore her hair. The maiden hairstyle of a *maiko,* called *wareshinobu,* was characterized by a bagel-shaped, rolled knot worn high on her head, decorated with ribbons, ornaments, and silk flowers. A less decorated style with the knot lower down, called *ofuku*, meant the *maiko* had had her first sexual experience.[20] A small lock was pulled back tightly for the *maiko* hairstyle. Over the years this fell out and did not grow back, creating a little bald spot on the crown of the head. Older geisha proudly show off this "*maiko* medal of honor."[21]

Courtesans also had a "hair ranking system," which varied over the centuries. In earlier eras, the simpler the coiffure, the higher ranking the courtesan. In later times, a *tayu* could be distinguished from a lesser-ranking courtesan by her ostentatious hairstyle sporting numerous "needles" and combs.

Hair Tips
- In modern Japan, daily bathing is an important ritual, and this includes washing your hair. Japanese women use shampoos rich with nutrients and with such ingredients as rice bran, olive oil (brought to Japan by the Portuguese in the sixteenth century), and dried seaweed to remove dirt and excess oil.

Azuki Bean Soup to Banish Dark Circles under Your Eyes

Ever notice how smooth the face of a geisha is, even under the eyes? No dark circles for her. What is her secret? *Azuki* bean soup is a favorite tradition that helps to diminish the appearance of dark circles around the eyes by cleansing your body from within. Small, dark red, and oval, delicately flavored *azuki* beans are a good source of energy and help lower cholesterol.[h]

- Soak 3 cups of beans in a large pot of cold water for 24 hours or overnight. Drain.
- Add 2 quarts of cold water with the beans to the pot and bring to a boil.
- Drain the beans, then add 2 quarts of fresh cold water again.
- Simmer for 30 minutes, then add 2 Tbsp. of cumin and 1 Tsp. white pepper.
- In a frying pan, sauté the following ingredients in 1 Tbsp. of olive oil until tender: 2 diced carrots, 2 Tbsp. of fresh ginger, 3 cloves of garlic (minced), 1 large, sweet onion.
- Add the ingredients to the soup, then cover, and simmer for 30 minutes, or until beans are cooked through.
- During the last 15 minutes only, add salt to taste (otherwise, the beans become hardened).
- Just before serving, add juice of 1 fresh lime and 3 Tbsp. of fresh cilantro.

- Japanese women are fond of massage for health and relaxation. They know that proper hair and scalp hygiene includes cleansing *and* stimulation; a foot massage or hot footbath can also aid poor circulation in the head area.[22]

HANDS

Hands are an important part of every woman's seduction repertoire. The hands of a geisha soothed a man: " . . . each touch of her fingers was a motion produced by long practice. It was poetry of the hands . . . [that] flowed into a harmony of action, sound and color. It unfolded itself like a flower under the morning sun."[23]

The geisha used her graceful hands to pour tea, hold a fan in the correct way (with her thumb inward and not showing), or arrange a flower. Lifting or touching something "just so" shows respect and transmits a feeling of importance to every action.

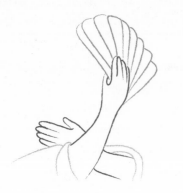

The hand motions practiced in dance added grace to everyday movement

Hand Tips

- In Japan, a woman's hands reflect a certain grace of movement even if she is not a trained geisha. She practices using her hands properly.

- Hand lotion is essential to Japanese women, especially during the cold weather. She protects her hands from the elements by carrying an umbrella and, when wearing a kimono, folding them into its long sleeves.

- Hands should be clean and well-groomed. Massage them by pulling the skin back toward your wrists. Don't forget your nails.

- Character and personality are reflected in your hands; a class in *ikebana*, flower arranging, or *chanoyu*, tea ceremony, as well as taking a dance class can help you learn how to use them gracefully.

FEET

In Japan, the feet are an essential element in feminine beauty. Courtesans went barefoot even in winter.[24] In Ihara Saikaku's novel *The Life of an Amorous Woman* (1686), a young girl who is being appraised as a possible courtesan for a high-ranking official is described in this manner: "Her feet were scarcely eight inches in length; the big toes were bent back, the arches elegantly raised."[25] Geisha used their feet with restraint and grace, mostly because of the kimono, which instructed the body directly in the feminine art of walking, sitting, or standing.[26]

FEET TIPS

- Even your feet are part of the act when you make love, so you want them to be beautiful. Maintain them well. Bare feet with well-trimmed toenails, tinted red, were the ultimate of chic among late-eighteenth-century Fukagawa geisha.[27]

- Follow the Japanese custom of removing your shoes when you are in your house and wear slippers indoors to relax your feet.[28]

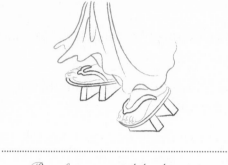

*Bare feet represented the ultimate in
chic for the Fukagawa geisha*

- The sensual Japanese woman also knows the importance of *shiatsu* foot massage to balance her internal organs.

Luxuriantly glossy hair, beautiful eyes, flower-like mouth, exquisite hands, and graceful feet—these made a pretty courtesan, but by themselves, they didn't add up to one with *hari*, spirit. That could only come if she had also mastered the remaining points of *kokono-tokoro*, those subtle hints of something smoldering within.

POSTURE

"Have no fears, my beautiful one," he whispered. "You draw all eyes and hold them so that they see naught else. You will dance tonight like the Moon of a Thousand Ripples—like the cherry blossom in the morning wind! Remember, you will be dancing for me. It may be years before I see you with my eyes again, but the memory of this night will live with me till then."

Mrs. Hugh Fraser, *The Heart of a Geisha*, 1908

The curve of her form suggested the grace of a wind-blown willow, the designs on her robe promised the arrival of spring, and behind her small red mouth awaited a wealth of possibilities to fulfill every man's desire. For the geisha and courtesan, graceful movement was a natural part of their repertoire. Is your body movement graceful?

A seductive presence begins with the physical poise that comes from a good body image. How can you believe your man loves your curves if you don't love them yourself? Don't hide under the sheets. Self-confidence is the most seductive trait you can acquire. That was why a courtesan did not retreat bashfully when someone approached. Instead, she "cast glances," *nasake-mezukai,* even when she did not know a man, turning around carefully as she passed in order to make him think she had fallen in love with him.[29]

The geisha was extremely careful about posture, knowing it to be basic to a slim, trim figure. Wearing a kimono with a stiff *obi,* "sash," around the waist, ensured she would stand straight, chest up, stomach in, and hips aligned properly. Geisha also developed perfect posture and graceful movement through the mental and physical discipline of rigorous dance training. You can attain that kind of mind-body balance with exercise and meditation. Combining the two will help you gain flexibility, breathing control, and stress relief for your mind as well as your body. A toned body is a comfortable body. Joints that don't hurt move gracefully. You can also improve your body image by eating a proper diet and drinking plenty of water.

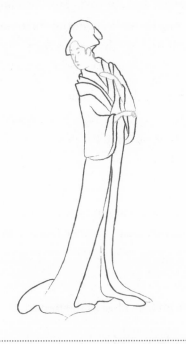

The geisha exemplified perfect posture, accentuated by the folds of the kimono

POSTURE TIPS

- Western dress allows more freedom of movement than kimono, but body awareness is just as important. Take a ballet class and you will discover that every movement a dancer makes is centered in the hip or pelvic area.

- You can encourage good posture by doing the following exercise to properly position your pelvis: Stand tall, back to the wall, feet approximately two inches from the baseboard. With your spine touching the wall, slide your torso down to a sitting position, hold, then push yourself back up the wall to your original position. Do five to eight times daily.

- Geisha sleep on the floor on a futon, with firm back support beneath provided by a *tatami*, straw mat. Try sleeping on a firmer mattress than you are used to doing and you will notice the difference in your posture. Practice sitting: Do not back up to a chair and drop into it. Instead, keep your spine straight, then lower your torso from your hips and sit gracefully into the chair. Or into his lap.

- Japanese women never cross their legs for a long period of time. It is bad for circulation. Always sit with your stomach pulled in, knees parallel, feet together.

SEDUCTIVE AIR

. . . fragrance rose from the cushions and from her robes as she moved.[30]

Even into the twentieth century, travelers to Japan were fascinated and enchanted by the delicate physicality present in the women of the pleasure quarters, as you can see in this excerpt from a 1933 travel journal: "Then she sank back on a pillow, balancing herself, as

Flowers and Japanese Women

Heian ladies, courtesans, actresses, dancing girls, bathhouse girls, and geisha were portrayed as exquisite creatures, feminine ideals likened to flowers, as in the poetry of ninth-century femme fatale Ono no Komachi, where she described the beauty of a woman with the phrase "the color of flowers."[i] Ihara Saikaku also referred to women as flowers when he wrote, " . . . a flower endowed with the gift of human speech," meaning an intelligent woman.[j] The word for flower is *hana*. Consequently, the phrase *kaigo no hana*, "word-understanding flower," was used to describe the great beauties of his day. Even as late as 1927, the poet Hagiwara Sakutaro wrote, "Geisha were truly the 'flower of civilization' of the Edo period."[k]

Geisha took these words to heart and used them in describing their professional status. The areas where geisha worked were called *hanamachi*, "flower towns."[l] The fee paid for the services of a geisha was called *hanadai*, "flower money,"[m] or *ohana*, "honorable flower," in the geisha community.[n]

she did so, almost on her fingertips. It was a curious aesthetic movement delightful to see."[31] It was not only the pretty young geisha or courtesans who possessed this seductive air, the older women also had the same power: " . . . then she [*mama-san*] folded elegantly to her knees, propped her chin on her hand, tilted her head, and looked provocatively out of the corner of her eye. Suddenly one could see . . . the grace of her movements . . . she could have any man on his knees."[32] This is your objective.

"SEDUCTIVE AIR" TIPS

- When the geisha entered a room, she was never rushed or out of breath. If you want to make an impression on an entrance, remember, "poise" is almost synonymous with "pause." Giving yourself a moment is a chance to relax, and plan what you are going to do and say. Diaphragm breathing can help you relax: To the count of five, inhale deeply through your nose; also to the count of five, exhale through your mouth. Make sure your shoulders don't move; if they do, you are not breathing correctly.

- The power of graceful movement made the geisha or courtesan seductive, whatever her age. You can become more graceful by practicing in front of a mirror: Shake your hands briefly to relax them, and note the way they naturally fall: fingers set apart, forefingers extended. This is the basic position of a dancer's hands.

- Every word, every action should convey your personality and femininity. That's why a geisha accented her gestures with a fan or a small parasol. Used with skill, a pair of sunglasses or even a ballpoint pen can be a prop to create a teasingly seductive air to your movements, and also convey something specific about you.

- *Maiko* wore six-inch high clogs with tinkling bells called *okobo* to add to their height. "Wedgies" or high heels will arch your foot, give you height, and also create a more graceful line that makes you appear slimmer. High heels are also sexy, whether you are wearing clothes or nothing at all.

- Traditionally, geisha bathed together in public bathhouses. Get used to being nude: Walk around the house *au naturel* or take naps in the buff.

- What is *not* seen has a seductive air all its own: In the days of Old Edo and long before, just the sight of gorgeous robes caused great excitement and sexual desire: " . . . unworn garments on racks inspire the viewer to imagine their appropriate owner—usually a beautiful woman."[33] Their air of mystery even inspired a sensually evocative type of screen painting called *tagasode byobu*, meaning "whose sleeves?"

Sex is as much about the visual aspect of lovemaking as the act itself. The way you move can enhance what he sees in a big way, especially the way you walk.

YOUR WALK

When she went on procession to a rendezvous, an Edo courtesan walked with a suggestively rhythmic and voluptuous gait known as "figure eight" walking[34] or *ukeayumi*, "floating walk," swaying her hips loosely and throwing out her feet as though she were kicking up something with the tips of her toes.[35] Arriving at the teahouse, she entered with a "skipping gait," *tobiashi*; she entered a hall soundlessly with *nukiashi*, an "exposed gait."[36] So distinctive was this walk that artists of the time alluded to it in their renderings of these women, using what is called the "Kano school line," a calligraphic style that gave an animated, curvaceous sensuality to their drawings.[37] Geisha captivated every man with the glamour of their seductive walk, leading one writer to rhapsodize, " . . . gliding in [the room] on the soft cat's-paws of their white stockinged feet, it made me think of evening clouds."[38]

The courtesan was well aware that physical beauty may start with your figure and posture, but motion brings it to life. The way you walk, the way you sit and stand, the way you move your hands, these are things

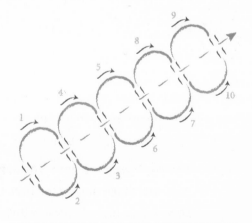

The slow "figure eight" step pattern gave eye-catching rhythm to the courtesan's walk

that make your beauty count. The first time he sees you, you may be sitting and eating, or talking on your cell phone, but in most cases you are entering a room or walking across it. It is by your walk that he will gain his first impression of you. What will that impression be? Will he see a woman of grace?

WALK TIPS

- Make your walk graceful, light, and smooth, with good posture. Keep your buttocks tucked under, hold your stomach in, stand erect and tall, and hold your head up and back.

- Work on achieving natural motion in your arms, swinging them forward and back instead of holding them stiffly at your side.

- Plant your feet as wide apart as your hips, distributing your weight evenly. Bend your knees as you walk and rotate your hips with each step, shifting your weight from side to side.

- Stride by leading from your thigh. The length of your step should be about three-quarters the length of your foot. Longer steps will make your stride masculine; shorter steps, mincing.

- Keep your weight evenly distributed on the entire foot, not the balls alone. Let your heel touch the ground first, while taking the next step. With each step, you contract the muscles in your buttocks, which is the motor that drives your walk.

- If you want to turn heads like the courtesan in her high *geta,* wooden clogs, with her sexy, va-va-voom walk, wear high heels.

A courtesan knew that all eyes would be on her at all times, even when climbing the stairs. For that, she had a special, delicately hurrying step, *hayameashi*, and never cast her eyes downward.

CLIMBING STAIRS TIPS

- Don't throw your weight forward with each step or allow your body to tilt downward as you descend. It is awkward and clumsy and your waistline disappears, making you look heavier than you are.

- Don't rush. As you take a step, hold your posture position, your head high, and your buttocks tucked under. Don't hold onto the railing.

- Practice stair walking while wearing a sexy teddy and high heels and nothing else. Don't be surprised if you have an audience.

VOICE

Voice is often overlooked in the art of seduction. Even the sexiest words won't turn a man on if the sound of your voice grates on his ears. Sensual Japanese women have known for centuries that it is not only words that seduce, but also how you say them.

That is why a geisha included voice on her list of essential arts. Kyoto geisha even had their own dialect with unique expressions replacing the usual words for such things as "kimono" and expressions like "excuse me, please."[39] Every geisha's voice had a sensuous quality to which she devoted years of training, "vigils during winter nights when the geisha pupil had to practice her singing on the roof under the stars, till the cold broke her voice and gave it the wild hollow note which is sweet in Japanese ears."[40] The result was a strange yet compelling sound, at times "somewhat coarse and also more flexible, thus enabling her to sing the traditional songs"[41] as well as "soft and lilting."[42] Men found it all irresistibly charming.

I am not suggesting that you spend the night hours on your balcony singing to your neighbors; instead, have a tape recorder running as you talk on the phone, chat with friends in your home, and read aloud from a book or magazine. Then listen to it. Be objective. Signs that you need improvement: if what you hear is high, squeaky, whiny, or weak; if people tell you that you sound like a little girl; if you are very loud or speak very fast; if your sentences are endlessly interrupted with "ums" or "like"; or, simply if you are embarrassed by how it sounds to you. Never fear. With a little practice, your voice can create that important first impression and make him want to hear more.

VOICE TIPS:
- Many women believe a "low, husky" sound is seductive. Be aware that speaking

at the very bottom of your pitch range can result in problems from strain. You want your sound to be seductive, but natural.

- At the other end of the spectrum, very often "singsong" or whine patterns appear when you are under stress. Loosen up by reading out loud to him from a sexy, erotic novel, and don't forget the sensual sound effects.

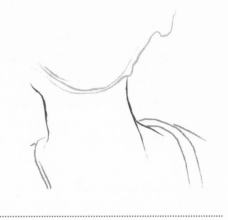

The nape of the neck is considered especially erotic when exposed to view by a low collar

- When speaking, pay attention to the bridge and sides of your nose, down to and around your lips. Voice experts call this area the "mask" because ancient Greek actors amplified their voices with masks worn over this part of their faces to focus the sound. A voice emitting from this area will be open and flexible, expressive and warm, with a resonance that will both impress and seduce.

A FINAL THOUGHT ON SPIRIT . . .

The essence of the sensuality of the Japanese woman can be summed in the word *hari*. Yet *hari* is not determined by a woman's physical appearance, age, or station in life. It is defined by an indefinable toughness of spirit. Higuchi Ichiyo, a woman of letters in Meiji Japan, said it best when she came upon such a woman:

A geisha . . . a heartbreaker, no doubt. . . . "She must have made the thrushes cry," as the saying goes. She has not completely lost her beauty . . . someone who's experienced enlightenment . . . she thinks rather highly of herself. . . . The woman bears paying attention to.[43]

And so will you.

Chapter 2

BATHING PLEASURES

Bathing once, the visitor was made fair of face and figure; bathing twice,
all diseases were healed; its effectiveness has been obvious since of old.

Izumo Regional Chronicles, A.D. 733[1]

In the same manner that you wash your hands before dinner, the geisha and courtesan washed their bodies before going to a banquet or to bed for an evening of sexual pleasure. In Japan, the bath remains a way of life. Ninety percent of Japanese take a bath at least every other day.[2] Bathing promotes good circulation, helps cure insomnia, reduces stress, and strengthens and improves your skin. But more than that, the simple, sensual pleasure of bathing can connect your physical, emotional, and psychological well-being to revitalize your spirit *and* your body for sex.

HISTORY OF THE BATH

Almost all Japanese institutions come from China, but the concept of cleanliness is original with Japan, where bathing has always been both a physical and spiritual cleansing. As part of her daily ritual, the geisha went to a shrine to pray. There, she rinsed her mouth and hands at a fountain placed there for this purpose, according to the Shinto belief that personal dirt is disrespectful to the gods. Priestesses in ancient times took this belief one

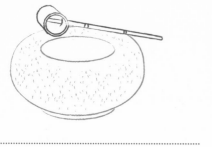

....

A basin and ladle are used to cleanse the hands
and mouth before important ceremonies

step farther. When they ventured on religious journeys to the sacred Inner Ise Shrine, they took part in the purification rites of *yuami* and *misogi*.[3] They also bathed nude in an icy cold stream or under a waterfall before entering the shrine,[4] refreshed and purified, their senses alive with an invigorating excitement. At the end of *hadaka matsuri*, "naked festivals," you are washed of your impurities in a river, lake, or the sea. These festivals also revere the showing of sacred objects. Isn't showing your body to your lover also a spiritual and stimulating experience?

The Japanese have known about bathing pleasures for centuries and make *ofuro*, the "honorable bath," an integral part of their lives. *Sento*, community bathhouses, existed in the cities of Kyoto and Kamakura even in ancient times. In the early Edo period they prospered, employing young women called *yuna* who enticed customers with the lure of sake and a hot bath, where they assisted men in and out of their clothes and in combing and doing up their hair in the *chonmage*, top knot, that was the custom. It wasn't long before these bathhouse girls began doing more than running their fingers through a man's hair and offered "special services" in the steamy rooms. These establishments were often disguised brothels since the *yuna* were less expensive than prostitutes. In inns, *hasuha-onna*, "lotus leaf women," and *ashisasuri-onna*, "legstrokers,"[5] who attended to travelers, were known for not being deeply committed to chaste conduct.[6] Ordinary women in the towns had their own lively and sensual interludes in bathhouses in their "floating world bath," often bathing next to geisha, who took public transportation to the bathhouses in Tokyo.[7]

While the sexes often bathed separately, mixed bathing also existed in both cities and countryside until a law passed in 1900 prohibited such mingling. But, except in the large cities, the public didn't pay much attention. In the country and at *onsen*, hot spring resorts, the sexes continued to bathe together. This notion of bathing *au naturel* is most likely the source of the phrase used to refer to the closest friends: *hadaka no tsukiai*, "naked acquaintances."[8]

While it is true many Japanese "do not see" bath time nudity, they are discreet in using the towel, not only as a washcloth but also as a fig leaf. This "nude togetherness" often startles foreigners, but as J. R. Brinkley, historian and editor of the Yokohama newspaper *Japan Mail* remarked many years ago, "The nude in Japan is to be seen but not to be looked at."[9] Nevertheless, back in the late nineteenth century when ladies wore bustles, Western women in Japan entered hot spring baths clad in dressing gowns or cotton kimono to avoid the embarrassing act of "exposing their bodies to curious eyes." This led to the misconception that Europeans had tails, since the Japanese interpreted the bustle as an apparatus solely for the purpose of enclosing the woman's tail, coiled-down when not in use.[10]

The stones of the entrance to a *ryokan*, traditional Japanese-style inn, are ritually washed as an act of purification and also as a sign of welcome. You are purifying yourself when you wash your body as you prepare to welcome your man. It all begins with your bathroom.

BATHTUBS

The ideal Japanese bathroom is not the cold, metallic, tiled place common to inns and public baths. Instead, it is an extension of the bath itself. Everything possible is made of that warm, comforting, restful substance, wood. And this means tubs. Most Japanese prefer tubs

Ocean-scented Seaweed Bath

To revitalize your skin, combat stress and fatigue, boost your metabolism, and eliminate toxins, prepare a bath made of edible seaweeds: *kombu, wakame,* and *funori.* These edible seaweeds are loaded with protein, iodine, amino acids, and vitamins and are available in leaf form or in more convenient prepared packets. Sprinkle powdered seaweed directly into bath water heated to 100–107 degrees Fahrenheit, then soak for twenty minutes. After bathing, wrap yourself up in a thick, fluffy robe, then lie down under a silky quilt with your head and feet raised up slightly on soft pillows. Relax for twenty minutes, then shower and scrub your body to stimulate cell activity and circulation.[a]

of *hinoki,* cypress. When warm, it gives off a delightful pine-like scent. The traditional tub also can be hand crafted from chestnut, Chinese black pine, or cryptomeria. Japanese tubs are shorter, but deeper than what you are used to, and often have a built-in seat, made for a deep, soothing soak. Three broad planks make a lid to keep it hot until ready.

Even an ordinary Western bathroom can be *your* place to be on your own. A bath should be your own special time to unwind, de-stress, and think your own pleasant, sexy thoughts. Turn your bathroom into a spa-like sanctuary. If a Japanese-style wooden tub does not appeal to you, another adventurous approach is the spoon-like sculpture tub fashioned in porcelain. Make your bath pure enchantment by adding Japanese touches to your bathing area such as *yuzu* (yellow citron), green moss, dewy gray rocks, a leafy potted plant, a scented candle or two, and your favorite relaxing music. Muted colors, soft natural light from your garden outside or lowered lights, along with water sounds and the whiff of subtle plum blossom or pine incense, all induce serenity. Before you get into the bath, pack a basket with a scrub soap or shower gel, bath oils, bubble bath, bath mineral salts, and body lotion. You are ready for bathing pleasures.

HOW TO TAKE A JAPANESE BATH

In Japan, you wash your body *before* you soak in the tub and relax. You sit on a low bamboo stool, or you can scrub in the shower. To begin, you need a small wooden bucket, a natural bristle back brush, a pumice stone for the rough spots on your elbows or knees, a small absorbent washcloth, a scented bar of soap, shampoo, and conditioner. Soap up, washing your underarms, feet, and genital areas, scrubbing your elbows, knees, the soles of your feet, and your back. Rinse thoroughly with water ladled out from the tub, or in the shower. Your body is clean. A *tenugui*, a linen cloth about the size of a small guest towel, traditionally serves for both washing and later, drying, but fluffy Western-style terrycloth towels also are a delight. After you wash your body, you climb into the tub and wash your soul.

Bath water is for soaking and relaxing, and is very hot. Varying anywhere from 95 to 140 degrees with an average of 107.6 degrees Fahrenheit, the water seems much too hot at first. Add bath salts to help prevent dizziness and the extreme fatigue sometimes caused by hot-water bathing, and also for a refreshing or soothing fragrance. Prior to immersing, douse your body and head repeatedly with water from the bath or rinse in the shower, until you feel warm all over. Five to ten minutes will enable you to adjust to the heat more easily. Then get into the bath. Let yourself slide down by sections— legs, waist, and breasts. Sink slowly up to your chin. Move as little as possible when you first

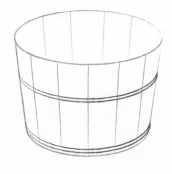

A traditional Japanese "hot tub" is made of cypress and is designed for soaking

Sake Bath

Fill your bathtub with hot water, then add one to two quarts of sake. Soak in the *sakeburo*, "sake bath," for at least thirty minutes to smooth and soften your skin. This is an antitoxin bath that goes back at least three thousand years. It has been suggested the ladies of the Heian court enjoyed it for its enhancement of beauty.[b]

get in, or you will feel the heat more. If you remain still, you can stand high temperatures. Soak until your pores open and the sweat starts rolling down your face and body.

This is your time to relax. Thinking about your problems defeats the goal of releasing your stress and fatigue. Use this time for meditation, although meditation in the bath takes practice. Empty your mind of worldly distractions. Lean back; let a drop of water fall, and watch as it creates circles on the surface. Close your eyes and focus on a word or phrase, like *mu. Mu* means "non-existence." For now, nothing exists except you and the bath. Breathe slowly, deeply, as you repeat *mu.*

After soaking in the tub, step out on the tiles. Don't stand up suddenly when you emerge from a hot bath: Dizziness and fainting are common dangers. Douse your head in cold water. Then either do as the Japanese do and remove excess water with your damp *tenugui*, or dry your body with a fluffy towel.

AFTER YOUR BATH

Slip into a loose-fitting cotton kimono, called a *yukata*, and lie down, wrapped snugly in a blanket for the same amount of time you spent soaking in the tub. This will allow for maximum benefits from your hot bath. Your rest period can be followed by a warm-water scrub, a cool shower, and the application of oil or emollient all over your body. Think sexy thoughts while applying oil to the erogenous zones of your body and you will be surprised how good it feels.

BODY SCRUB AND SEAWEED PACKS

As you sweat in the tub or in the sauna, a wide range of toxins stored in your body fat and blood are excreted through your pores. Detox baths with baking soda, Epsom salts, or sea salt can also help eliminate toxins from your body. Soak for fifteen to twenty minutes, then scrub your skin gently with a soap brush made from a natural fiber, such as a boar-bristle, dry brush, or a loofah mitt.

Salt rub treatment makes you glisten like the sparkle on a geisha's silver hairpin. Try dry skin brushing, an old natural healing method used by geisha, to increase blood and lymphatic circulation. Brush your whole body once a day with a natural-bristle dry skin brush found at health food stores. Use short, brisk strokes, always brushing toward your heart for maximum benefit.

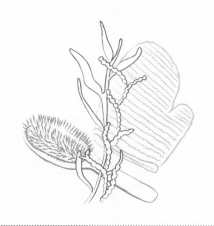

A loofah mitt, brush, and seaweed can be used for a detox bath

The seaweed body pack is a regenerating, revitalizing, and cell-activating treatment that brings extraordinary sparkle and tone to your skin. Use *wakame* seaweed. Fresh *wakame* should be soaked briefly in warm water, then rinsed to remove the salt. Dried *wakame* must be soaked for twenty minutes for softening. After thoroughly scrubbing and cleansing, apply the seaweed strips all over, or on those areas where you would like to appear especially sexy. Then recline for thirty minutes. Remove the seaweed, rinse off with cool water.

Ginger compresses (consisting of a topical application of fresh, hot ginger water) dispel cold, stimulate circulation, and assist your body in the breakdown of fat deposits.

SPAS

Shinto, one of the two main religions of Japan, has always attached the highest importance to ritual purity—and this includes the bath. Buddhism, the other religion, regards the body as nothing but an illusory outer covering and not to be noticed. Combine the two and you have . . . nude group bathing. Where else is nude group bathing more appealing than in the numerous *onsen* resorts?

Picture a beautiful pool of clear, hot mineral water lined in dark gray rocks and surrounded by volcanic vents that spew up jets of pungent, sulfur-laden steam wafting and billowing from the water. The scent permeates an *onsen* town. The Japanese believe mountain water is therapeutic for your spirit. For centuries it has called both geisha and samurai to speed the healing process, whether it was a broken heart or broken bones. A hot bath at a *ryokan* often uses hot spring water fresh from the mountain. Treat yourself to a sybarite's delight by visiting one of these retreats. There you will learn what you can do to rediscover the natural rhythms of your body through rest, healthy diet, sunlight, and fresh air.

This steaming symbol on maps and signs indicates the presence of a relaxing hot springs

Although in most *ryokan* each room has its own small bath, large separate-sex and communal baths offer once-in-a-life-time experiences. The bathing area may be constructed from stone or wood, and many bath choices are often available for your pleasure: hot or cold, milk or lemon. A traditional sulfur bath will leave your skin feeling like silk. An outdoor bath, called a *rotenburo*, is located in a scenic spot. You take your *tenugui*, go to the bathhouse, and leave your clothes in a wicker basket. Don't be surprised if everyone is naked. Sharing the enjoy-

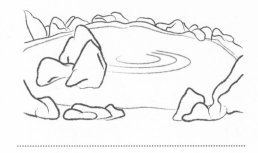

Outdoor baths in a scenic location are perfect spots for romance and relaxation

ment of beautiful mountain or forest scenery while soaking in a steaming bath is uniquely refreshing, especially with that special someone.

If a trip to an *onsen* is just a dream, you can set up your own retreat in your home. Portable spas can provide therapeutic benefits in the privacy of your backyard. The massaging action is created by sending a combination of warm water and air through jet nozzles, resulting in an "energized" stream of water that loosens knots of tension in your body. It relaxes your tired and aching muscles, eases arthritis pain, induces restful sleep, and increases mental relaxation and acuity. Many modern Jacuzzi have a unique bowed design with contoured armrests and a sloped backrest that fits into the style of any bathroom. Soaking in hot water laced with soothing fragrant bath salts, surrounded by lovely flowering trees and shrubs, you can have your own *rotenburo*. Do as the geisha did in the *sento*. Hum a tune as you scrub, soak, scrub, then soak again. You take on the glow of an added sensuality as you submerge in the hot water, your breasts glistening, your tummy flatter, your hips sleek and trim. When you emerge, body and spirit are cleansed; your troubles and fatigue—and old relationships—are rinsed away with the dirt.

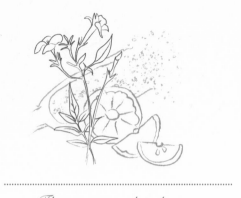

Flowers, citrus, and rice bran can all be added to scent the bath

Geisha folklore suggests that water offers health and preserves youth and, according to ancient beliefs, some hot springs seem to have special healing and rejuvenating powers. One is the *wakasai*, "well of youth," at Nara, where in the coldest days of winter the priests of Todaiji gather to draw water in a ritual called *omizutori*. You can enjoy this same ritual by installing little fountains of water in your home and office and experience firsthand the soft, inner rhythm of water that has given the Japanese culture its ability to let go and to flow.

BATH SCENTS

One of the most important items in bathing Japanese style is the addition of flowers and scents. Your bath may contain flowers (iris, rose, chrysanthemum), leaves (daikon, carrot, cherry, peach), fruits (citron, tangerine, orange), roots (lotus, ginger, iris), or rice products (sake, rice bran).

Bath Scents Tips

- Make your own bath salts with pure essential oils, salts, and pretty bottles. You can find salts with such fragrant names as blackberry sage (blue/purple), bubble gum (pink), eucalyptus mint (light green), mango sage (light orange), and Hawaiian white ginger (white).

Yellow Chrysanthemum Bath

You will need edible yellow chrysanthemums. Float the flowers in your hot bath. Soak, but do not rinse. It is probable that the courtesans of Yoshiwara indulged in this warming, youth-giving bath to keep the ravages of age at bay.[c]

Citron Bath

This enchanting bath gives off a delightful, feminine fragrance. Use dried citron peels or whole fresh fruit (lemons can be substituted). A variation on this bath is the citrus bath to improve circulation and ward off colds. Slice any kind of citrus—limes, lemons, oranges, or grapefruit—and float them in your hot bath water. If you like, you can substitute dried peels for fruit. You can also use tangerine or mandarin orange peels or whole fresh fruit for an aromatic and spirit-soothing bath that perfumes your skin. Break dry peels into small bits then tie them into a piece of gauze, and fasten it with a cord. Place the bag, or four or five whole tangerines if you prefer, in a hot bath, then soak.

Rose Petals Bath

Use ten roses, plucking the petals (after they have been sitting in a vase for a few days), and scatter them on the surface. Almost immediately, moist, perfumed air rises from the water, giving you a relaxing bath. Keep the water temperature a bit lower than usual to preserve the rich rose color. You can also put rose petals in a diaphanous cloth bag before adding them to your bathwater to save time cleaning the tub.

- For hydrotherapy baths, use sea salt, algae, clay, mud, or essential oils.

- For muscle relief, use oils like lavender, rosemary, eucalyptus, chamomile, juniper, peppermint, camphor, bay, and ginger.

- For a deeply relaxing bath, select bergamot (an uplifting herb that smells like oranges), chamomile, lavender, marjoram, mandarin, rose, or sandalwood. Do not use more than four different oils per blend.

What About the Toilet in Your Bathroom?

Toilets have come a long way. No longer just functional necessities, they can be a part of your relaxing, cleansing routine. Modern toilets offer new luxury and comfort with gentle aerated warm water, self-cleaning dual-action spray, a quiet, soft-closing seat, and a heated seat with temperature control. They are easy to install and offer you the ultimate in cleanliness, including dual action front and rear washing. They also offer massage with back and forth water cleansing, a dryer with three temperatures, a deodorizer to remove unwanted odors, as well as remote control.

TAKING A BATH TIPS

- Don't bathe within thirty minutes of eating, since the effects of hot water interfere with your digestion. The best time to bathe is when you're not very hungry and you have time to dream.

- Welcome yourself to your special bathing place with a cup of green tea, scented candles, and a steaming facecloth rolled up like a scroll.

- The sensual Japanese woman uses a *hechima* (loofah), a *nuka-bukuro* (silk bag filled with rice bran; see chapter 1), and a *karuishi* (pumice stone).[11] You can find similar items in a bath store to enhance your bathing pleasure.

- Drink a glass of water, juice, or tea thirty minutes before bathing to provide necessary hydration to induce sweat and open pores. You can rehydrate your body after your bath by drinking a glass of cool water.

- Save drinking wine for after your bath (and after drinking water).

In Japan, no bathhouse is complete without a *sansuke*, masseur, to scrub your back and massage your tired limbs. Next, you will explore how massage can help you become more seductive.

MASSAGE

Massage, the use of touch and various manipulation techniques to move your muscles and soft body tissues to relieve stress, tension, and pain, is a therapy going back four to five thousand years. One of the earliest books on Chinese medicine, *The Yellow Emperor's Classic of Internal Medicine,* written in 2700 B.C., lists massage as a treatment for paralysis, chills, and fever. More than likely, the Japanese used this chronicle to perfect their own unique type of massage: *shiatsu. Shiatsu* is a popular acupressure technique that focuses on "rebalancing energy." The therapist's fingers apply strong, rhythmic pressure along points on your body, including your arms and legs, to reduce tension from stress. In macrobiotic *shiatsu,* the meridians on your body are massaged by the thumb, hand, elbow, or foot pressure of the masseur, giving you the resulting benefit of regulating and balancing the capacity of your organ systems. *Shiatsu* massage can also be sexually arousing if you—or he—hit the right spots.

Although massage therapy does not cure disease, it does promote a sense of contentment and relaxation. When your muscles are overworked or strained, whether from exercise or from trying out new sex positions, waste products accumulate and cause unpleasant spasms. Massage helps by improving your circulation, bringing more oxygen to those areas through increased

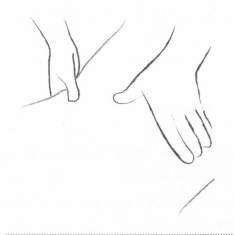

After your bath, a massage can be
sensually and sexually arousing

Soothing Bath Tea

Try this lemon lavender tea. You will need one-half cup lemon balm, one-half cup lavender, and boiling water in a quart container. Steep ten to twenty minutes, then add to your bath water. Add a few drops of essential oil of lavender, diluted in a quarter cup of neutral oil (such as almond, sunflower, or walnut), to your bath water for an extra relaxing plus.

blood flow. This accelerates the elimination of waste products from your body, promoting healing—and your sexual well being. Massage reduces your heart rate and lowers your blood pressure. It increases the release of endorphins in your body, the same feel-good chemicals as from an orgasm. Massage is also credited with reducing pain and depression and helping to improve the overall quality of your life. Often, all it takes is a simple touch to lessen the stress and anxiety of a long day. A good massage can leave you refreshed and energized and ready for sex.

MASSAGE TIPS

- Follow a warm, soaking bath with a hot-stone massage, using smooth basalt stones.

- Geisha of Old Edo enjoyed the touch of a blind masseur, not to hide their nude bodies from glances, but because they believed massage done in the dark made it even more relaxing. Ask your man to give you a massage in the dark and you will discover a new meaning to the phrase "touch me all over."

- *Do-in* is a self-massage technique said to increase your circulation and digestion as well as strengthen your muscles, organs, and nerves.

A FINAL NOTE ON BATHING . . .

A luxuriating hot bath is not pampering, but a valued and essential part of your sexual life. Do as the Japanese do: Relax and take your time. It is considered bad taste to hurry while bathing. While you are in the bath, don't forget to meditate about him. In the next chapter, you will learn the technique of *erotic* meditation.

Chapter 3

EROTIC MEDITATION

At midnight, your face in a dream brings a sigh.
Ch'u's love pavilion was long ago far away.
But like a blossom on the flowering plum,
Sweet narcissus blooms between your thighs.

Ikkyu (1394–1481), Zen master[1]

According to legend, the beautiful woman in this charming poem was Lady Mori, a blind minstrel and the favorite mistress of the sexy Zen master who wrote it. She embraced the arts of seduction to evoke a state of erotic meditation in the mind of her lover. Meditation has been used for thousands of years to find inner peace and nourish the soul. In this chapter you will explore how to find your inner sexuality through erotic meditation, using breathing techniques, diet and sleep, the benefits of tea, relaxation methods, and the art of masturbation.

WHAT IS EROTIC MEDITATION?

Contrary to some popular beliefs, relaxation is only superficially what meditation is about. Meditation will slow you down with a healthy reduction in heart rate, blood pressure, adrenaline level, skin temperature, and stress hormone levels, but lulling yourself into blissful semi-consciousness is not your ultimate goal. You aim to elevate your mood to a heightened sexual awareness, making a perfect prelude to an encounter.

The goal of all meditative procedures is to quiet and focus your mind outside a judgmental framework. The goal of erotic meditation is to release any sexual shame or discomfort you may have and increase your pleasure and openness to love. It is an inner journey to heighten your amatory senses, to intensify consciousness of your body, mind, and emotions, and to experience them as a unity as they relate to sex. Being intensely aware when you are *not* having sex enhances the experience when you *are*, because you learn to be "in the moment" whatever you're doing, whether you are preparing for sex, having sex, or resting in his arms afterward. Meditation ultimately enables you to manage your sexual energy into a positive flow and regulate your emotions.

How do you begin?

Set aside a specific period each day to meditate. Put it in your daily planner as your time for solitude, listening to your inner self, and reflecting. Do as geisha did and indulge a part of you that always feels stressed and tired: Put a pair of clean white socks into the dryer for a few minutes, then put them on. Their warmth around your feet will help you relax and unwind. Then, in a quiet, private space on a comfortable surface such as a mat or carpet, lie down and elongate your spine, or sit upright with your spine straight,

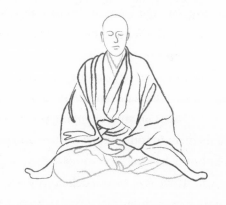

Seated meditation can help you relax and extend your openness to love

either cross-legged on the floor or in a firm chair with both feet on the floor. With your eyes closed or gently looking ahead, take in a deep breath through your nose, all the way down to your stomach, and exhale through your mouth. Observe the exhalation of your breath but don't obsess over it. You are ready for erotic meditation.

The point of meditation is *not* to soar above your physical self, but to come to know and accept the entirety of your personal reality, especially your body. Whether or not all is perfect in your eyes now, with awareness you can come to understand how your mind and spirit relate to your body, and that together they create your unique physical beauty. What the world sees is an outer manifestation of your balance with nature and your harmony with the universe. You understand and enjoy your femininity and sexuality as part of this beauty. This frees you of any aversion to being naked before a man.

To take this point one step further, too often you dream about the perfect date based on a past experience or fantasize about an experience yet to happen. Instead, live in the present and enjoy this moment, this night, with a lover. By helping you find yourself as a natural part of the universe, meditation not only forces you to concentrate on the here-and-now, but also helps you recognize and appreciate that in life, even your sex life, there is nothing *but* change. As part of a natural order, your last orgasm won't be like your next, and so on.

Focus on your changing physical sensations: How soft your breasts feel when you touch them, how your nipples harden and get pointy when you pull on them, the roundness of your buttocks when you squeeze them together, how easily your vagina becomes moist when you stroke it or have a deliciously sexy thought, or the innermost contraction you feel below your pubic bone when you tighten those muscles. The goal is to bring the activity of your mind in perfect sync with your body, "being in the zone," as they say. If your mind wanders, simply acknowledge it and return to your "out" breath. Imagine your thoughts as if they are clouds dissipating away, like the floating world. Serenity is important. This is part of your spiritual life.

Meditation is paying attention to what you are doing, whether you're sitting quietly out in your garden smelling the flowers or thinking about the hardness or softness of a lover's body. It is connecting in a personal way with whomever or whatever you are focused on. Spend time thinking about the

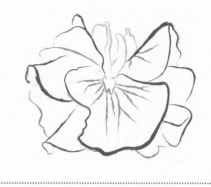

Use a beautiful flower as a starting point for meditation

things that bring you peace, harmony, beauty, and calmness. Geisha spent time appreciating the beauty of a single flower, a butterfly in flight, a gorgeous sunset, or the feel of a silken kimono between their fingers, and so should you. Making love will be one of those things when you come to know it in this way.

BREATHING

Geisha are known for their beauty and their ability to create serenity in everyone they meet. What is their secret? Their inner calmness is due to proper breathing.

Breathing is synonymous with life. Inhaling and exhaling are involuntary, automatic actions controlled by your brain. When you are born, the first thing you do is inhale. After that, you typically take twenty thousand breaths a day without thinking about it. Although your lungs can hold two gallons of oxygen, studies show you probably breathe in only two pints.

Let's take a look at how your lungs work: They are complex organs located within your chest cavity, inside your rib cage. They are made of spongy, elastic tissue that stretches and constricts as you breathe, bringing in fresh, oxygen-enriched air and expelling "used" air, mostly carbon dioxide. As you inhale, air is pulled through your windpipe, past your vocal cords. It enters the bronchial passageways leading deeper into your lungs. The air continues its race through narrower and narrower tubes in your lungs called *bronchioles* until it reaches the *alveoli*. These are grape-like sacs where oxygen and carbon monoxide are exchanged in and out of your bloodstream.

Tension causes you to experience shallow breathing. Deep abdominal breathing therefore counters stress, sexual or otherwise.

According to some experts, your nose has the advantage in breathing, especially outdoors, because it is a natural filter. Nose breathing results in deeper breaths than mouth breathing, filling your lungs into the lower lobes. Nose breathing also stimulates your *beta-endorphins*, the hormones associated with calm and a sense of pleasure,[2] putting you in the mood for love and all *its* pleasures.

Others say it is better to breathe through your mouth to help your body take in more air. Nose or mouth, suck in the air and breathe. The point is to get the air into your lungs whatever way works best for you.

BREATHING AND SEX

When you are exerting effort, as in having sex, the demands of sensual activity interrupt your normal breathing rhythm. Deep breathing exercises consciously intensify this natural physiologic and sexual reaction. They can be very useful during a stressful situation, especially if you are concerned about impressing a lover with your sexual expertise or if he is worried about *his* performance. The solution: Taking a deep breath is an automatic and effective technique for winding down or preparing for the "tease" in sex. It is also useful for maintaining a relaxed state until you are able to let yourself go.

Deep breathing also keeps you focused in the moment and helps you deliver enough oxygen to your lungs and, consequently, to your bloodstream and muscles. It will help reduce tension in your body and make a sexy movement less difficult—and a fantastic orgasm easier to achieve. When you breathe properly, your body functions more efficiently in every capacity—including your sex organs.

Mindful, erotic breathing takes practice. As you inhale, feel your chest and stomach expand; as you exhale, feel your stomach shrink. Remind yourself to check your breathing often during sexual activity. It helps to take deep breaths even when you are not in the frenzy of having sex. Try it when you're giving him the once-over in the supermarket or eyeing that bulge in his pants over cocktails. It may be just what you need to de-stress while you enjoy the view.

TEA

Green tea has been a staple of geisha and courtesan lore for centuries. Drinking it aided the complexion. (In modern times, we know why: Green tea contains *polyphenols*, strong antioxidants that protect against cell damage to the skin.) When they were young girls, these women were taught to perform the tea ceremony to attain poise, grace, and confidence. In Japan, the expression "you have tea" is used for someone who has mastered the tea ceremony beyond its rules, rituals, and procedures so that it has become second nature. The phrase can also refer to a woman who has mastered the art of life. For example, you could tell by the way a geisha knelt and slid open the shoji screen when entering a room whether or not she "had tea." Without her speaking a word, her poise and elegance made it obvious that she

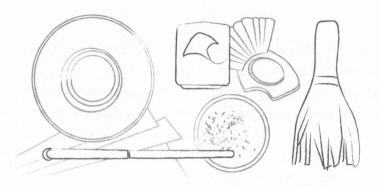

A bowl and whisk are just a few of the traditional utensils used in the tea ceremony

had entered a place of freedom, effortlessness, and grace within movements practiced numerous times. Study the graceful gestures of the tea ceremony and you will understand why it brings out not only the artistic essence of life, but also a sensual awareness that is part of erotic meditation, like tasting the frothy, bright green tea with its slightly bitter flavor of spring grass, *shunso* (also an old Japanese term for pubic hair).[3]

HISTORY OF TEA

Tea comes from *Camellia sinensis,* an evergreen shrub native to China. According to legend, an emperor discovered tea over five thousand years ago when the leaves accidentally fell into his cup. The Zen Buddhist monk Dengyo Daishi is believed to have introduced tea drinking into Japan from China in A.D. 805 and, with it, the Chinese word for tea: *cha.*[4] Originally monks and priests drank green tea as medicine and as a stimulant to aid study and meditation. Eisai Zenshi, a Zen priest, returned from China in 1191 with *matcha,* a vivid green powder of ground leaves.[5] Out of this grew the tea ceremony, a spiritual art best known as *chanoyu,* or *chado,* "The Way of Tea."

In the tea ceremony, the preparation of *matcha* is a form of meditation. Performing the tea ceremony for a lover can be one of life's nicer moments—the savoring of a unique place, time, and relationship between you and him. As with anything worth doing, there is a certain style, training, and many rules to follow that when fully mastered will bring you to that "Zen zone." So should be the preparation for, and the end result of, making love.

The tea ceremony is about finding order, balance, and harmony within yourself and with those you have invited to share the experience. It celebrates the aesthetic beauty in the mundane, the superiority of spirit over matter, and tranquillity within busy lives. The traditional tea ceremony begins when you enter a small thatched-roof hut along a garden walkway. Its spare, simple interior expresses *wabi,* understated elegance. Stooping to enter, you shed all worldly pretensions and take on a reverent, humble attitude. In an atmosphere of ritualized preparation, carefully scripted movements allow you to enter a state of deep concentration. First, you eat seasonal sweets, then you sip the frothy, bright green tea, using beautiful bowls and utensils chosen with great care and thought for that occasion. Your senses are awakened and sharpened by the sounds of rippling water steaming in the kettle, as well as the delicious contrast on your tongue between the tea's slight, grassy bitterness and the intensity of the sweets, and by the beauty of the objects and setting.

A full tea ceremony takes four hours, not thirty seconds like the Western tea bag dipped into hot water. To do properly, it is a discipline that takes years of practice. But you can approximate it in your own space. Clear your area of clutter and choose a comfortable mat to help you relax. Keep your décor simple, selecting "cool" tones such as green, blue, or lavender. Add scented candles and low light (avoid direct overhead lighting) to bathe you and your guest in shadowy warmth. You can also add elements of nature to add to the spiri-

Types of Tea

There are three basic types of tea: black, green, and oolong. What distinguishes them is the process by which they are made, that is, the treatment of the leaves.

For green tea, the leaves are steamed or pan-fried, which prevents oxidation and allows them to retain their green color. It has a delicate, clean taste, a subtle aroma, and a beautiful pale green color. Black tea is made by fermenting and roasting the leaves, which gives it its characteristic dark color and rich taste but also destroys some of the nutrients contained in the plant. Oolong, a brown, mildly bitter tea, is only partially fermented.

Flavored teas combine pure, natural flavors with fine black tea leaves. Fruits, flowers, spices, and natural flavors are added to the tea to create exciting and exotic tastes and aromas.

Herbal tea does not contain tea leaves. It is an infusion made from flowers, herbs, fruits, and spices. It is packaged and brewed like real tea and yields an array of delicate, subtle flavors and aromas.

tual ambiance. Use soothing sounds such as a miniature fountain or a CD playing nature sounds. You can also add water to your space by filling a bowl and floating delicate pond-weed on top. Add an aromatic shrub and small stepping stones to complete your at-home *chashitsu*, tearoom.[6]

A SENSUAL APPROACH TO TEA

The tea ceremony is a journey in which the senses are a vehicle to quiet the mind. Each moment is one of deepening awareness. The sensations of taste, hearing, smell, and touch become more intense. You and your partner are part of this focus, becoming closer and closer until your souls come together. Your separate existences dissolve. You understand sexual life, including loves past, present, and future, as an element of nature, and the ecstatic sounds of love as reflections of nature's life force.

So also are the good and bad moments, which you accept like the sweet cookie before the bitter tea. As a meditation, the tea ceremony encourages balance and putting your mental "house" in order, and this includes your love life. Just as participants bow in a gesture of thanks, you and your lover should show each other courtesy and respect. You spare no expense on items used in the tea ceremony. You should spare no expense to take care of love in your life. Green tea is said to aid longevity and good health. What more do you need?

Tips for Getting the Most Benefit from Green Tea

- Green tea retains chlorophyll, and with it, many healing components. Use it on skin to soothe sunburn, swelling, and itching, as a disinfectant for acne, and as an after-shampoo rinse once a week to add luster to your hair.

- Drink two to five cups a day to receive its therapeutic effects. It has only fifteen milligrams of caffeine as opposed to eighty-five milligrams in a cup of coffee.

- Cleanse your breath by chewing on rehydrated leaves.

- Tea leaves can be simmered, steamed, smoked, and stir fried, or added to recipes as a spice.

- Drive away mosquitoes by burning dry tea leaves in a pot.

- Ensure good sleep, promote clear thinking, and improve your mood with a pillow filled with dried, used tea leaves.

WA, KEI, SEI, JAKU

The tea ceremony relies on four important concepts that can be your guides in your sexual life. *Wa* means harmony. With careful coordination of the accoutrements and décor, you create a harmonious and sensual experience. *Kei* is the respect that you show for each other in moments of physical intimacy. *Sei* is purity. The cleansing of your body, mind, and soul before sex represents the detachment you have from worldly concerns and the orderliness that should govern your life. *Jaku* is tranquillity. You can achieve this calmness through the constant application of the first three principles in your everyday life. Create a sanctuary where the two of you can take solace in the tranquillity of the spirit to experience the most satisfying sex.

FROM TEA TO ZEN AND BEYOND

Think of tea, and you think of Zen. They are like fraternal twins, so closely related, but very different. The tea ceremony awakens the senses in an atmosphere of ritual and discipline. Zen meditation is not confined to a formal practice. If you are fully present, Zen happens: while washing your hair, applying your deodorant, or getting out of bed. It can happen when you make love. This was the lesson of the famous monk Ikkyu, who after years of study in the monastery, found enlightenment in sake, in poetry, in fine food, and in the brothels of Kyoto. He knew that only with discipline can you become truly free. Then you are truly naked. Sex is only about the body unless you can become open and as aware of your partner as you are of yourself. This takes time. Allow yourself to get lost. There are no goals or intentions. Just . . .

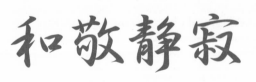

Tea concepts: wa (harmony), kei (respect), sei (purity), jaku (tranquillity)

MEDITATION AND ZEN TIPS

• Draw up the sheet and blanket, letting it

Improve Your Sex Life with a Better Diet

As part of her training, the *maiko* got up at a certain time in the morning and performed her ablutions, greeted the other members of the household, said her prayers, then ate her breakfast.[a] More than likely this occurred within one hour of waking, which was critical to how her metabolism worked for the rest of the day.[b] Missing a meal because you think you will look slimmer in your new, low-cut dress leads to low blood sugar. A physical drop in your blood sugar can cause emotional anxiety.

Stabilizing your blood sugar levels may mean consuming four to five small meals a day rather than three big ones. Eat foods low in fat and sugar, as the geisha did. The sushi (red shellfish, squid, tuna, cucumber roll), *tempura* (shrimp, pumpkin, vegetable), *miso* soup, *wakame*, tofu, pickles, noodles, and rice of the traditional Japanese diet have little if any refined sugar. Eat fresh foods rather than processed, served in small portions.

cover your body with coolness. Feel the warm water trickling down your neck, your shoulders, your back while you wash your hair. Listen to the sound of the water and say, "Ah."

- Put on your makeup foundation and feel the silky wetness. Look at your reflection in the mirror as you apply it. Touch your cheeks, feel the width of your nose, the curve of your chin, and the softness of your lips.

- Clean your house or apartment before a lover comes to spend the night. Cleanse your personal space of anything that will distract from a night of great sex and romance.

- Japanese women have special days when they pay respect to old bras, needles, and other ordinary items. *Harikyu,* "needle mass," is when needles broken in service are put into a cake or block of tofu and set to rest. Give items one moment of respect, one moment of thanks, and one moment of thought.

- Listen to soothing music on headphones, covering your eyelids with an aroma-therapy eye pillow scented with a few drops of cucumber or lavender essential oils. Take a deep breath, and on the exhale, feel the releasing tension.

- Focus awareness on your face and feel it release tension. Do the same with your neck. Take your time. Continue downward to your shoulders, breasts, back, arms, fingers, abdomen, thighs, calves, feet, and toes. Imagine a door at the bottom of each foot. Arch your foot and open the door and let tension exit, then squeeze your toes downward and close the door. Repeat.

- Pop the cork on a bottle of champagne, spilling it all over each other, then lick it off his face.

- Feel his hardness with your fingers when slipping a condom over his penis.

- Picture a pleasant and relaxing place. It can be imaginary or real. Take yourself there, feeling, smelling, and hearing the sensations of the place.

SLEEP

The geisha, courtesan, and hostess are called "Butterflies of the Night" because they don't go to bed until the early hours of the morning. Getting adequate sleep is one of their most important beauty secrets.

You should average seven to eight hours. Sleeping in after a night of wild, exciting sex is fine, but if you sleep too long, it throws off your body rhythms the following day. It is better to go to bed earlier the next night, especially after your hot bath. If you don't get enough sleep at night, daytime naps can be invaluable to maintaining an interesting and

Japanese Gardens

When it comes to erotic meditation, Japanese-style gardens have an allure all their own. The idea behind a meditation garden is to escape the world and its distractions for a purer place where, surrounded by the calming influence of nature, your imagination can transport your mind into a higher sphere. It is designed to express the fleeting, impermanent quality of beauty and of life itself. Don't expect bright colors or heavily perfumed flowers. Color is sparing, just enough to add interest to an atmosphere of monochromatic green. These natural greens relax your eyes, producing a very serene effect. Plants are chosen for leaf shapes and textures: broad-leafed taros and callas, heart-shaped water lilies, sword-like iris and flax, and an edging of rambling, prostrate juniper. A meditation garden can also be composed of boulders and gravel, raked in interesting patterns so the shadows play upon the stones. The sun, the moon, and the rain give the stones different, constantly changing subtle colors and textures, sharing an inner harmony that obeys natural rhythms and fills the garden with energy.

The objective of a Japanese garden is to idealize nature rather than regiment her. You will find stepping-stones, gates, stone lanterns, and *tsukubai* (hand-washing basins). You may also encounter floating bridges crossing a stream rushing down a tall granite sluice lined with small stones, flowing into a gentle creek that appears and disappears under flagstones before vanishing. The garden can be set among a grove of redwoods, wild grasses, or black pine trees and various bamboo. Every step you take reveals something as it hides other elements. Go out late at night and lie next to him under the trees and look at the moon.

What do these quiet, reflective places have to do with erotic meditation? They are visually and sensually seductive, and reveal themselves only slowly. Think of your body as a garden as you reveal to a lover the swell of your pretty breast, then conceal it, then reveal your bare midriff or navel. It is this new inner confidence achieved with erotic meditation that makes you so seductive.

robust sex life. Keep them short, five to twenty minutes. A nap lasting longer than thirty minutes can make you feel groggy. Naps help your mind, body, and soul get back to where they belong, and also boost your creativity.

Sleep can be part of your erotic meditation ritual, if you focus on remember-

Mint

Mint can help you prepare your body for erotic meditation by easing indigestion and combating fatigue. More than twenty-five varieties exist, including chocolate mint, lemon mint, orange mint, pineapple mint, apple mint, and even banana mint. The oldest known variety is *Mentha x piperita*, peppermint. Peppermint and spearmint are both available in the United States. All contain menthol, a component of the volatile oil that gives the plant its characteristic smell and flavor, and peppermint has the most.

Highly aromatic, mint is a refreshing addition to most foods, including cold drinks, hot teas, baked or broiled fish, etc. It combines well with garlic to flavor meat and lamb and complements cilantro in salads; it is also an excellent addition to desserts that feature ginger, lemon, or chocolate. Mint stays fresh in the refrigerator much longer than other herbs. It also may be frozen or dried. To store, wrap in damp paper towels, then place in a sealed plastic bag and refrigerate.

ing your dreams. Are you having "wet dreams"? It's possible. Dreams are soul-nurturing and orgasm-inducing, often satisfying a sexual longing unfulfilled in daily life. Dreams are communications from deep within that represent where you are on your path of spiritual growth, and also help to guide you onward. Daydreams also are healthy, a kind of erotic meditation if you let them wander freely. Light a candle in the bathroom and take a bath. Or, go outside, lie on the ground, and stare up at the sky. Get a silky kimono and wrap yourself in it for an extra-sensuous feeling.

MONO NO AWARE

The ladies of the Heian court spent much of their day contemplating nature and writing poetry that expressed an emotion they called *mono no aware.* This was the exquisite, deep, epiphany of feeling prompted by the experience of extreme beauty: Its briefness revealed the transience of all things. Though plaintive, it came from an intense awareness and sense of intimate union between the poetess and nature, or between her and her lover—or between you and yours, to drink in the glory of a summer day, wander down familiar gardens, or play with the *koi* fish in the pond.

You can experience a kind of *mono no aware* by appreciating each moment what you love most about him: The way his right eyebrow lifts when he's sexually aroused, his cute butt, the hardening of his penis when he presses his body against your belly, and the musky smell of him after sex. These are moments that are all the more special because they are brief. Do this when you're alone. It is a form of meditation you can do anywhere. Take twenty minutes where you will not be disturbed. Choose a comfortable position, sitting or lying down, and make certain your clothing is loose and comfortable. Take off your shoes and say, "Ah."

Don't get too relaxed! Next, you are going to explore the ultimate in erotic meditation: Masturbation.

MASTURBATION

Shunga, "spring drawings," the erotic art of the Edo period, often show women in the act of masturbation, whether it was with a leather dildo or the protruding penis-shaped nose on a mask. There was no shame involved in the art of masturbation. Neither should you feel any. Masturbation is the first natural sexual activity that you experience. It teaches you body awareness while you engage in self-touch, and it is the ongoing love affair you have with yourself throughout your lifetime. It can help you maintain and strengthen your inner physical health and to prolong orgasm and intimacy. If you usually reach orgasm only by clitoral stimulation, masturbating with your finger or a sex toy can help you discover the pleasure of a G-spot orgasm, a technique enjoyed by geisha, who employed a dildo to achieve sensual pleasure.

Sex is less about being nude and worrying about breast size and more about how you manage the erotic life energy within as it builds and pulsates between you and your lover. From the beginning of her training, the geisha used masturbation to learn the sexual skills of conscious breathing, body movement, and visualization that took her out of her head then back into her body. It is an erotic meditation that can help you increase your sexual enjoyment *and* control, and teach you to release the fear, anger, and internalized repressions preventing you from experiencing your full erotic power. Here are some tips to help you.

MASTURBATION AS EROTIC MEDITATION TIPS

- Set aside some time for yourself. Don't let daily life invade these love-sessions. You will find you look forward to these dates with yourself. And yes, even if you have a man, you may still wish to masturbate, especially if you're in the mood for sex and he's not. The wise courtesan knew that you should never place your sexual satisfaction completely in someone else's hands. You are in control of your sex life.

- Next, set the mood. Dim the lights, burn some erotic incense, put on some soothing *shakuhachi* flute music, spread out a futon as the geisha did when the teahouse was quiet, put on a loose-fitting kimono *sans* panties, make sure you have some white tissues, and set out your favorite sex toys and lubricant.

- Masturbation inspires creativity within you. Loving yourself allows you to design these occasions of your sex life as if you're an artist with a living canvas. Put a drop of lubricant on your finger and apply it to your clitoris. A drop is all you

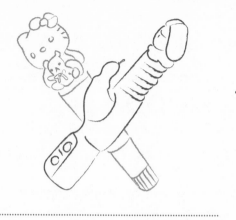

Vibrators are instruments of personal pleasure and come in all sizes, styles, and degrees of whimsy

need to glide to ecstasy as smoothly as the geisha glides across a polished floor.

- Prop a mirror in front of you as a guide. Observe your clitoris, then your urethral opening, and if it moves when you insert a lubricated sex toy. Don't be afraid to feel inside, then to slide your finger into your vagina. The more you know about your body, the sexier you will feel when you make love.

- Don't rush. Masturbate slowly, taking all the time you need to become aroused.

- Don't rely on fantasies to achieve sexual pleasure. Instead, focus on your deep breathing and being relaxed, keeping in the mind the serenity of the geisha as she explored her physical feelings with her dildo. You can do the same to release your blocked emotions and achieve greater spiritual connectedness and inner peace.

You have the right to peace of mind—whether you find it in erotic meditation or masturbation, herbs, or a cup of tea. When you feel your body and mind connect through meditation and deep breathing, you will feel a great sense of release. Knowing this, imagine what kind of sexual release you will feel the next time you make love with him.

In the next chapter, you will set the sensual mood for a night of passionate lovemaking.

Chapter 4

INTOXICATING MOOD ENHANCERS

Everything takes on greater beauty at night: our attire, the décor of a room, or the magnificence of ceremonies . . . at night perfume and music most fully reveal their exceptional attributes.

from *Idle Hours* by Urabe Kenko (ca. 1330–35)[1]

The sun rose as the third-century warrior empress Jingo Kogo rode her stallion through the cold, white, snow-covered Kitayama cedars to meet her lover. Or did she fly by magic over a profusion of red, red maple leaves rustling in the warm wind? Or, in a moment of passion, lie with him amid the delicate flutter of falling pink cherry blossoms? All three scenes evoke different yet sensuous moods. In this chapter, you will learn how to involve all of your erotic senses to create the perfect romantic atmosphere.

If you fancy the James Bond type complete with English accent and Oxford education, make the room elegant and refined with pale hues of ivory, taupe, mauve, and gray, along with faux marble, nickel-finish brass, Tuscany accessories, and tapestry fabrics. If your imagination leans toward Indiana Jones, earthy, environmentally aware, and sophisticated, decorate your bathroom and bedroom with green. Use plants and naturally woven wood accessories, and interesting, exotic accents from foreign cultures. If you look for quirky and fun "frat-types," mix turquoise and marine blues with yellow, orange, and red, and use tropical designs for decoration—like you in a hula skirt with a lei around your neck and wearing nothing else.

Setting the décor is only the beginning. Let's get down to the basics of mood. Way down. Chemistry, smell. Human pheromones. These odor-rich substances are made up of certain chemicals that are similar to male and female sex hormones and that trigger distinctive brain activity when sniffed by the opposite sex. Scientists believe that a part of your brain involved in regulating sexual behavior lights up when you are exposed to a substance similar to testosterone. The same brain area in your man lights up when *he* is exposed to a substance similar to estrogen. This shows that the right scent is essential to seduction.

The Japanese know how important scent is to creating a mood, especially in your home. Geisha teahouses were cleaned daily, the futon aired out, and the rooms dusted. This tradition was wise. Particles and gases in the air can irritate your lungs as well as smell unpleasant. Be mindful of dust, mold, and household chemicals, including heavily perfumed toiletries, and rid them from your home. A seductive, romantic mood begins when you get to work and literally clear the air: Slip your hands into something comfortable such as linen polishing mitts. Use all-natural cleaning tools such as silk dusters, china twill cloths, flour sack towels, turkey feather dusters, horsehair brushes, and corn brooms. These steps reduce your exposure to indoor and outdoor air pollution.

And don't forget the bathroom. It doesn't have to be a dirty job, not with toilet cleansers and dish soaps scented with plant-derived essential oils that smell like jasmine-lily, lemon verbena, and rosemary-grapefruit. These products cost much more than those using synthetic fragrances. However, in addition to being healthier, they are pretty; the translucent emerald, amethyst, and amber-colored liquids in clear plastic bottles make charming window-ledge decorations.

Your home is clean and smells good, too. Let's decorate for a sensual mood.

DÉCOR

Arriving at an elegant *geisha-ya,* geisha teahouse, the visitor was escorted to *tatami* rooms graced by the relaxing sounds of a trickling fountain and decorated with low tables. He was asked to sit upon silk cushions with his back to an alcove called the *tokonoma*, the position of honor. The elegant guest would appreciate the hanging scroll or floral display, and have the manners to say so, as well as comment on the choice and arrangement of art objects. The hostess would bow and offer tea; it was correct etiquette to accept a second cup.

What does this have to do with décor? Simple. Everything in the *geisha-ya* had a proper place *and* meaning to ensure the correct outcome of the visit. When you invite that special man to your home, you also wish to ensure the desired outcome: lovemaking.

FURNISHINGS AND ACCESSORIES

If an interior designer arranges your home, it is called "styling." "House-fluffing" is the name given to the art of perking up your home by being your own interior arranger.[2] Give your home a makeover by changing the look of a room using only the things you already own and love; after all, these are the things that best express you. Move your piano (or have him help you, a lot more fun), rehang your artwork, and throw away dead plants. Hang beautiful old kimono on the walls; make a collage out of your favorite movie posters and party invitations. An interesting environment is a sexy one.

A sensuous décor is about the curve of your furniture, soft, luxurious fabrics,

Keeping Him Cool on a Hot Night

Geisha tolerated, even savored summer heat, by creating an illusion of coolness to divert their senses. A cast-iron wind-bell with a slip of stiff paper dangling from the clapper caught the slightest breeze in the doorway of the teahouse. Entry curtains, *noren*, made of crisp, gauzy hemp or other bast fiber, often light in color, moved gently. Paper butterflies added whimsical charm. The sound of water splashing on green bamboo leaves in a stone basin suggested coolness.

flattering lighting, and pleasant but evocative scents. Surround yourself with serenity, harmony, and beauty. The clean lines and modular design of traditional Japanese furniture have a minimalist, uncluttered look that blends well with many styles, but any style you prefer is fine, so long as it is done *well*. To create your sensual décor, train yourself to recognize quality and tasteful placement of furnishings by doing as the geisha did when she entered a banquet, noting the teahouse decorations, the artwork, and the food. Texture, color, pleasing lines and proportions, accents, lush wood finishes, and patinas add up to a subtle, suggestive environment.

Create a Sensual Décor Tips

- Balance and proportion are paramount. Strive for unity to prevent a cluttered look, but don't be boring. Surprise his eye. A contemporary room will do well with a few antiques, and a Japanese motif will find visual relief with a few contemporary accents. Mix and match to add richness and sexiness to your décor.

- Pick a room's focal points, then add color and texture. There is great power in the number one, as in one great thing brought to life in a stage-type setting. It could be anything that commands attention. One large picture will unify an area busy with individual chairs and tables, or balance a window. Take a piece of beautiful crystal and display it on a pedestal, lighted to advantage. The backdrop should not interfere with your display. Busy wallpaper distracts. Most often a soft, solid color serves best as a background—though a bold color is in order if the object is pale.

- Group accessories for visual impact. Hang up several pairs of funky old sunglasses, arrange your favorite CD or book jackets, frame a collection of postcards from past trips, or mount old earrings on a silk-covered board and you have instant art. Odd numbers are more interesting than even.

- Choice of wood sends a message: weathered, dark-stained, and natural grains signal a homey, fire-in-the-hearth feel. Maple parquet and detailed door and window moldings provide elegance suggesting tradition and long-lost craftsmanship. Sleek-looking bamboo flooring, a natural, sustainable material, is modern and slightly exotic.

- Surfaces play a role. Stainless steel gives a cool, modern motif. Velvet, silk, and nubby textiles, twisted cords, and fabric walls covered in rich colors create a warmly sensual environment.

- Textured objects make delightfully evocative accents. Shells from the beach, a craggy rock, a rough piece of driftwood, the sleekest glass paperweight, a smooth marble egg, furry toss pillows, chunks of crystal—all naturally awaken the sense of touch.

- Black, very much a part of traditional Japanese décor, is a dramatic accent that can help anchor other elements in the room. It always works better than white, mixing well with textures and with natural materials like stone, copper, and iron. It fits in anywhere, from traditional to cutting edge. And it is very sexy—imagine draping your shimmering nude body over a black-lacquered coffee table. Is there any doubt?

- Avoid clutter. Don't have all your favorite pieces, artwork, and mementos out all the time. Traditional Japanese décor is sparing and changes with the seasons. You can do the same, storing what you don't need between times. It shows you pay attention to your surroundings and keeps them interesting, like you.

MIRRORS

Geisha teahouses were designed to turn out toward nature. In the warm season, shoji and wooden outside doors, *amado*, as well as sliding wall panels, *fusuma*, can be entirely removed, opening the rooms directly to the surrounding foliage, flowers, and trees. You can achieve a similarly open effect with mirrors.

Mirrors are wonderfully versatile. They bring light from the windows into dark interior spaces, creating the illusion of a more expansive, brighter area. Their reflections eliminate the sense of separation between rooms, visually enlarging a space. Mirrors add sparkle and life. You can raise the erotic pitch of your favorite sitting nook with a gilded mirror, a Japanese screen, and a sensually soft chenille throw in velvet.

JAPANESE SCREENS

Japanese screens are more than decorative fixtures. They can transform interiors. The sliding *fusuma* is both door and wall-like room divider. A *byobu*, folding screen, provides space

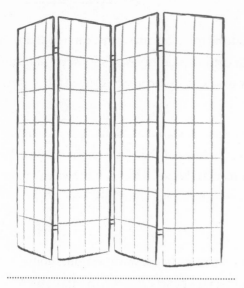

Japanese folding screens can be used to control light and intimacy in a room

definition and privacy, and is also used for ceremonial backdrops. Taken outdoors, it makes a temporary enclosure—wonderful for those nights of moon viewing and other sensual, nocturnal activities. Put a screen in front of your window. That way you can open it for some breeze and still have privacy during intimate moments.

The *sudare,* a curtain of reeds, is a popular summer screen. Or, hang up long lengths of thick bamboo joints and crystals strung on threads. The waving of these strings and their tinkling sound suggest the freshness of the stirring breeze; the crystals here and there are reminiscent of cool raindrops slipping down the bamboo stems.[3] Try walking through the curtain with your hips swaying. A definite turn-on for both of you.

YOUR BEDROOM

You will spend almost a third of your life in bed sleeping, unless you are otherwise engaged, so your bed and your bedroom are important. Evaluate the elements of your room for different sensual shapes and tempting textures. Add some organic element, a natural piece of beauty (besides you), such as fruit or flowers in a bowl or a glass vase, or mix them together for a succulent look. Look for interesting pieces to use as art, such as fans or pieces of kimono fabric. Place a minimum of three lamps or candles for flattering light. Think of what suits you and create a room that expresses it, whether it feels like a refreshingly cool sea breeze, or a warm and inviting cocoon.

Consider what you are sleeping on (not to mention whom you are sleeping with). Many mattresses need turning at regular intervals to keep their firmness and contour. Your mattress should smell and look invitingly fresh. Vacuum away accumulated dirt and lint. If there is a stain, use a mild soap and a small amount of cold water and rub gently to remove it.

There are many kinds and combinations of mattresses according to your preference, but you may find a luxurious featherbed mattress with a thick and fluffy mattress topper to be your ultimate seduction tool. A featherbed is not all about superficial indulgence. By cushioning and cradling pressure points like your hips and spine, it also positions your body in a comfortable and relaxing manner. No more tossing and turning (not, at least, when you're alone). Look for a filling of ninety-five percent feathers and five percent down, and a top layer of pure down. That "quill-proofs" the featherbed and achieves "loft," the plump resilience that looks so yummy and sexy. This is something you and your man can really sink into at night. What you do next is up to you.

COLOR

Color triggers emotions. Heian ladies, well aware of its sensual power, turned the multi-layering of colors into an art of intricate detail called *irome kasane.*[4] It has continued with variations and simplifications until recent times. This list of combinations is from the Ogasawara School of Etiquette.[5]

	NAME	OBVERSE	REVERSE
January	pine sprout	green	deep purple
February	red blossom	plum crimson	purple
March	peach	peach	khaki
April	cherry	white	burgundy
May	orange flower	deadleaf yellow	purple
June	artemisia	sprout green	yellow
July	lily	red	deadleaf yellow
August	cicada wing	cedar bark	sky blue
September	aster	lavender	burgundy
October	bush clover	rose	slate blue
November	maple	vermilion	gray green
December	chrysanthemum	lavender	deep blue

Make up your own chart matching colors that you like, traditional or modern: Electrified shades of watermelon, tangerine, and strawberry. A green more lime, less forest. Neon shades of blue, orange, pink. Mandarin orange and wild cherry. Cherry and plum blossom, wisteria from lightest to darkest purple, blue of iris, chrysanthemums of all colors, and the blood red of maple leaves. Use these colors in your décor accessories: hand-blown blue vases, notes written in passion pink ink, glass votive holders in go-go hues, accent pillows with splashes of color. The colors you like are the colors that describe you. Color makes you sexy. Don't be afraid to use it.

- "Dressing your walls" with color creates a perfect foil for your artwork. A transparent complementary glaze over a base color gives a soft, warm glow.

- Neutrals can set a romantic mood. All vary widely in tone, especially white, which can run from a warm cream to icy bluish-gray. Anything from a sun-baked beach to a shady forest to a tranquil horizon at dawn is a turn-on to most men. A room with a beige undertone always conveys warmth, and warmth in your home invites him to snuggle up close to you.

- Put your personal stamp on a monochromatic scheme by adding notes of richness and comfort with accessories like luxuriously detailed pillows. Add pieces in color schemes based in yellows, blues, or greens for effect. Pulsating, neon chartreuse greens create a trendy and youth-oriented attitude. Take advantage of texture in fabric, wall finishes, etc. to add extra interest in establishing the predominant mood.

- Be careful of very feminine colors like brilliant pinks, which are seen as whimsical and trendy. Although bright oranges are seen as gregarious, fun loving, and high-energy, too much of this color can be stressful.

- On the other hand, go for vivid yellows, which are seen as active and sparkling with enthusiasm and youthful vigor.

- Don't dilute the energy of the evening with subdued tones like lilac, sage, and periwinkle, colors seen as comforting, tranquil, and reassuring. You want to get him into bed, *not* put him to sleep.

Candles

The sight and scent of lighted candles infuse any room, especially your bedroom, with welcoming light and warmth, especially those with the fragrance of flowers: hyacinth and lemon grass, ylang-ylang and eucalyptus, rosemary, ginger, gardenias, or a wash of white roses. These are the aromas of dreams. Of desire. Candles summon the idea of romance and serenity. Fragrance candles come in jars, votives, wax potpourris, pillars, and tea lights. Pick your mood: vanilla or lavender for a peaceful atmosphere; pine and lime for an outdoorsy feel; or mango, pineapple, and melon for an island-like scene.

LIGHTING

In days of old, walking down tiny streets in the Gion district of Kyoto off the River Kamo, you were sure to see red paper lanterns painted with geisha names in black calligraphy swinging in the breeze outside the teahouses. Stop, and you could have seen rose-colored lighting behind the paper panes of the shoji and, using your imagination, its soft glow upon the faces of the beautiful geisha, the exposed napes of their necks, and their graceful hands moving through the air as they danced.

The right lighting is essential to setting a seductive mood. Shadows cast away from your face can add or subtract from your beauty, so evaluate your lighting well.

LIGHTING UP YOUR ROOM AND YOUR FACE TIPS

- Direct overhead lighting is "monstrous," casting downward shadows and giving a sunken-in-the-grave look to your face and body. Likewise, while blue is a calming color, the bluish tinge of fluorescent lighting is not flattering to your skin.

- Indirect lighting flatters. There are many options to suit any taste: wall sconces, table and floor lamps, controlled lighting such as inconspicuous low-voltage halogen recessed downlights and zenon linear cove lighting. All create wonderful layers of dramatic accent on your face and the rest of you.

- Photographers use orange filters over their cameras to give complexions a warm, healthy, seductive glow. You can get the same effect by putting them over your lamps. Your flaws will disappear.

- Candles create beautiful, dramatic lighting accents, but only when several or more are used. Depending on a single candle will give you a Gothic pallor.

- Directed lighting gives special objects in your décor dramatic presence. You can light an object from above, behind, or underneath. Test various angles with a flashlight to get an idea of which way the light best serves the object.

SKYLIGHTS

A favorite subject of many an *ukiyoe* is geisha and courtesans entertaining customers or playing games with each other on a teahouse open verandah. These women were well aware that natural light brightens your home *and* your mood. Make the most of natural light in your home by adding a skylight. Tucked into a vaulted ceiling or set atop a flat roof, a skylight allows light to pour into the interior spaces of your home from different angles, capturing sunlight throughout the day

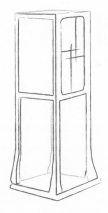

Floor lanterns fitted with candles or bulbs cast a soft and seductive light

in a way that warms and brightens the space. Even rainy day interiors feel more inviting. Create a glass-domed ceiling or skylight in your bedroom, and when it rains it's like making love under a waterfall.

Skylights provide three basic types of light: area lighting, task lighting, and dramatic lighting. Just illuminating an area is not enough. The ideal skylight clearly transmits light, with glazing eliminating UV radiation. This makes for a comfortable, beautiful interior that will set you off to advantage. It is important to know the location of the sun, particularly at midday and afternoon—and of the moon for your late-night moon-viewing parties. Consider what suits your needs, and how much light will benefit you.

SOUNDS

The bubbling of a fountain and the murmur of a garden streamlet falling from a bamboo pipe into a pool greeted all who entered through the gable-roofed gateway into the graceful, tranquil world that was the geisha teahouse. There, the seasons were defined by the soothing images and sounds of nature.

For over a thousand years, water has mesmerized the women of Japan and their lovers. They know well the mystical power of gardens, ponds, waterfalls, and streams to transport us from the hectic, ordinary world. The soothing sight and sound of moving water calms the senses and speaks to the fundamental needs of the human spirit—peace, and harmony. Without water, there is no life. It rightly sets the mood for lovemaking.

Music is also a powerful tool in the art of seduction. The geisha understood this, and she perfected her skill in the *shamisen*, three-string lute, and the thirteen-string *koto*, harp. What they knew from experience and instinct, science has now explained. Music rewires your brain, creating neural activities whose flashdance touches your soul. Your

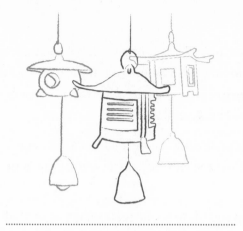

Japanese wind chimes have a delicate, resonant ring that "cools" on a summer night

brain maps the melody and forms a pattern. This dynamic map may hold the key to why listening to a certain type of music makes you feel like dancing or making love on one occasion but elicits a different behavior another time: as when you sigh, remembering those moments. Use music in this manner so the next time he hears "your" song, he will think of you.

To forge this sensual connection, the music must be harmonious with the mood you have created. Bluesy music for red lights and sheer black stockings; Chopin for pink lace and champagne; your favorite rock group for spiked pink hair and low riders; and country music for fringe boots, a low-cut gingham shirt, and cut-off shorts.

And don't forget the soothing, sensual music of the gentle wind chime, the *furin*. Geisha knew its clear, cool, otherworldly small sounds delight the senses. Its vibrations fill your soul with an enchanted, seemingly endless echo whose magical reverberations will remind you of an orgasm. Once you experience it, the memory never disappears.

SENSUAL SOUNDS TIPS
- Sometimes silence is music. Don't rule this out, especially if you are setting a romantic mood after you've both had a long day at the office.

- Music has the power of a mind-altering drug for a lot of people, but romantic or turn-on music is individual. Find out his tastes before your big evening, what artists he listens to, and his sensual favorites. Or, consider what you know of his interests and life to help you make your musical choice.

- Eliminate everyday noises such as phone, fax, television, loud clock alarm or pager, computer hum, or printer. You want to enhance, not distract, from your web of seduction

- Avoid loud music. You want your own sounds to be the most seductive and sultry of all, so don't let the background music or noise overwhelm you.

SCENT AND TASTE

The famed poetess Sei Shonagon wrote in her *Pillow Book,* "Things to delight the heart: Sleeping alone in a room tantalizingly scented with incense."[6] Japanese women have always known the lure of perfume—wafting in the air or permeating layers of silken robes. The aroma of a woman, be she geisha, courtesan, or Heian lady, lingered in the minds of her lovers. As one gentleman wrote: "I'd never consider it just an ordinary adventure to spend a night with you and then to leave at dawn, still bearing the scent of your perfume."[7]

The power of smell is one of your most important and evocative tools in the art of seduction. Many experts believe that smell has a more powerful impact upon your emotions than any of the other senses. A fragrance can transform your mood and make you feel sexy and romantic, sultry and naughty. It can transform his mood as well. Let's take a closer look at smell and see how you can use its power to your advantage.

HOW YOUR SENSE OF SMELL WORKS

A vestige of your primordial animal origins, smell stands alone as a direct link to your instinctual responses as well as your emotional life. What this means is that odor molecules, such as from perfume, body sweat, or the smell of sex, can dash right into the space in your brain occupied by emotions such as love and hate, and by moods such as anxiety and pleasure. Smell may actually account for more than ninety percent of the sense we call "taste." As you chew, tiny puffs of air containing odor molecules from the food follow a route that begins at the back of your throat and drift up the backward route to your nose. Add signals from the taste buds on your tongue as well as texture and temperature (something scientists call *mouth feel*), and you have "flavor." This is what most people mistakenly call "taste."

When your man snuggles up close to you and sniffs the freshness of your hair, bites on your ear, and tastes your skin, he also smells you. Each time he inhales, odor molecules, moving at lightning speed, race through the gateways directly behind the bridge of his nose to reach the *limbic lobe* of his brain, also known as the "emotional brain." Reaction to the smell comes first, even before he has identified the source of the odor. Scents also can affect your mood, sparking memories and experiences of memorable nights with memorable lovers. That is why a whiff of your perfume can send a lover adrift in a passionate paradise.

PERFUME

Your last date may not remember the dress you wore or your shoes, but he *will* remember your perfume. Perfume has that power to transform something ordinary, something everyday, into something magical. One drop can make you feel wrapped in the arms of your lover, transported back to a special moment you shared. Perfume is all about the magic of him catching his breath, of wanting to get closer to you, and keeping your memory in his mind.

From the Nara through the Kamakura periods (710–1333), small lacquer cases containing perfumes hung from a clasp on the kimono of an elegant woman. Later, the scent of a geisha was as personal as the stroke of her brush doing calligraphy. Well aware of how nature infuses flowers and plants with potent, seductive smells, she also knew the most important ingredient in choosing a fragrance was to capture the emotional essence and the spirit of the woman wearing it. *Your* scent should be just as personal, like your signature. Learn how to choose your scent, and use it to effect.

CHOOSING YOUR PERFUME OR FRAGRANCE

You are a woman and unique, and your perfume should convey that. Know the difference between an essential oil and a fragrance: An essential oil is the extract of a single flower, plant, or herb. Fragrances are chemical compounds. Good perfumes are made from combinations of the two. There are three main categories of perfume: Floral, Oriental, and Chypre. Floral perfumes are sweet, flowery, and suited to you if you tend to be happy-go-lucky. Orientals are powdery, sensual, and bewitching, and become those who like to show a little skin. Chypre perfumes are deep, oaky, and fit your style if you are sophisticated and tailored. In finding the right one, remember that subtlety and complexity are key to interesting scents.

To really know a fragrance, try it on your wrist, and wait ten minutes. The best fragrances are composed of multiple ingredients that "develop" on your skin, producing three effects: the "top note," your impression at the first sniff; the "middle notes," the blend of ingredients at the heart of the fragrance; and the "base note," the "dry down" aroma that lingers. If the base note expresses "you," this is your perfume.

Using Perfume Tips

- Don't try a myriad of different perfumes with your lover. Find the most provocative one or two, make them your only perfumes, and you, or at least the memory of you, will linger in his mind forever.

- Be appropriate. Warm weather enhances a scent, so switch to a lighter fragrance, like honeysuckle and jasmine with French lime blossom for spring, and to lime, basil, and mandarin grapefruit for summer. Use something light for daytime and save your heavy, musky concoction for nighttime seduction.

- To get the most out of your scent, put a small amount on your pulse points—the temples and base of the throat, as well as wrists, ankles, behind the knees (scent rises), the bend of the elbows, and between your breasts. Forget dabbing it behind your earlobes. The skin in that area produces an oil that diminishes the scent. He will never smell it when he is nibbling on your ears.

- Use restraint when applying a strong scent. No one should be aware of it beyond an arm's length from your body.

- Put scents in your refrigerator. When you spray or splash them on, they feel as good on your skin as they smell.

- Eau de toilette, short-lived but strong, is meant to refresh you. Eighty percent disappears in three hours, so don't reapply more often than every four.

- Perfume lasts twenty-four hours and has a softer smell. Even if you can't smell it, *he* can.

- With the exception of lavender, do not use undiluted essential oils on your skin and keep them away from your eyes.

INCENSE

The alluring sight of the beautiful Heian lady burning incense, *ko*, in her chamber intrigued the man spying from behind the lattice partition. He dared to come forward to watch closer. Using a rare *koro*, incense burner, she played the game of twenty perfumes with him: First, she sprinkled little black nuggets of incense in the shape of leaves, blossoms, or characters on the glowing coals, scattering green particles, brown particles, and grayish ones. Then she showed the gentleman how to catch the ascending column of pale blue smoke in his bent hand, closing his fingers upon it, and conveying it to his nose. The nobleman could not tell which he preferred, nor remember which dried particle gave forth a particular fragrance. Why? The incense, simply gums and resins in stick or cone form that give off scented smoke when burned, bewildered his nose with the commingled odors.[8] Bored with the game, he took leave of the lady for a rival. Use incense sparingly, lest your admirer become overpowered by the scent and take his leave as well.

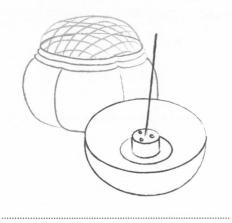

Incense comes in stick or block form and can freshen up any interior

Arriving in Japan around A.D. 500, the art of mixing and burning incense has a long history in formal entertainment,

Types of Incense

The fragrance of incense can reduce stress, ease depression, repel mosquitoes, and enhance meditation. Rosemary is often added to love incenses. It has long been known to increase memory, concentration, and even creativity. Modern research conducted in Japan confirms that it is a brain stimulant. An aroma session of rosemary and lemon will improve two lovers' concentration on what's most important.

Here are some other types of incense to improve concentration and get you both in the mood:

- *Aloeswood*, one of the most highly prized fragrances in Japan for its enrapturing aroma, is used to enhance meditation. The sensations gradually change from a faint, sweet smell to a feeling of peace and relaxation.
- *Citrus* of any kind is energizing and promotes an optimistic attitude.
- *Cloves* are an aphrodisiac and improve mental abilities, eyesight, and mood.
- *Frankincense* is spiritually uplifting.
- *Patchouli* promotes sensuality and a cheerful, peaceful attitude.
- *Pine* is a clean and refreshing scent.
- *Rose* promotes warm, loving feelings and peacefulness.
- *Sandalwood* promotes peaceful relaxation, is an antidepressant, and is spiritually protective.
- *Vanilla* is recuperative, physically energizing, and emotionally calming.
- *Violet* increases emotional sensitivity.
- *Ylang-ylang* is sexually stimulating and relaxing.

religious ceremonies, games, and no doubt in the art of seduction. Cinnamon, ground conch-shell, sandalwood, cloves, powdered herbs, plum pulp, seaweed, charcoal, and salt were among the ingredients mixed into pastes, then pressed into cones, spirals or letter-forms, and burned on beds of ashes. During the Kamakura period, certain woods were discovered to have more pleasing aromas and varying emotional effects when burned. Later eras saw an incense-stick clock that changed its scent as time passed, and another that announced the time according to one of several chimneys from which the fragrant smoke issued.

Scenting Your Personal Spaces Tips

- Scent the air with candles, a metal oil burner, a hanging ceramic container, cone and stick incense, or a copper lightbulb ring. When the lamp is on, the heat of the bulb perfumes the air.

- Create a fresh aura in your room by choosing from an array of new, refined aromas, such as citrus, herbal, woody, or garden varieties, including geranium, lavender, honeysuckle, and old rose.

- Make your bedroom more glamorous and appealing with the fragrances of heaven, romance, and sex: Patchouli, clary sage, heliotrope, geranium, rainforest, and English garden.

- Avoid "fragrance abuse." Scent should whisper, not call out across the room. Measure how much fragrance you use with your brain, not your nose. A little will entice, too much will send his senses reeling.

TASTE

Taste and smell, known as "the chemical senses," are far less developed in humans than in animals. Scientists believe this is because vision and hearing, which are processed through the rational side of your brain, the *cortex*, are more important in human society. In the strict sense, taste is limited to your perception of saltiness, sourness, sweetness, and bitterness, and the glutamate-inspired, deliciously savory sensation the Japanese call *umami*. All the other subtleties of flavor are combinations of these basic qualities plus your sense of smell. Perhaps that is why the enjoyment of food is such a many-layered thing.

A geisha never ate at banquets, but if she became an *okami-san*, teahouse owner, it was her responsibility to make certain the food served was of the highest quality both to satisfy the hunger and entice the eye of her gentleman guests. Japanese banquet food is more than rice and raw fish artfully arranged. It is more than simply the freshest and most perfect ingredients. It is redolent with meaning, of the season, the occasion, a poetic or erotic moment. Fortunately, our custom is to share a meal with a lover. We can learn from the geisha that a meal can be one of life's great sensual experiences, and a prelude of more pleasures to come. Isn't this the message you want to send to your man?

SEXY CUISINE

Imagine a meal that begins with a scoop of *toro* tartare, moist, raw, deep red tuna, topped with glistening, gray-green beluga caviar, awaiting you in a gleaming glass bowl. You spread the mixture on dominoes of bread, fragrant from toasting on the hibachi. The warm toast, fat-rich tuna freshly smelling of the sea, and the cool, salty caviar are a sensual, suggestive encounter of mingled flavors, texture, scent, and vision. This is a moment worthy of the most extravagant geisha banquets of the past, the *ozashiki*.

You can create your own banquet for two in your own home. All it takes is some preparation time, a few changes in your dining area, and a willingness to experiment. Let yourself go!

SENSUAL FOODS

While it is true that many Japanese foods border on the exotic, such as gold-flake-dusted

Bento

A *bento* is a "box lunch." It comes in a four-compartment, lidded lacquer *bento* box—the Japanese version of the picnic basket. The compartments offer so many interesting tidbits: meat, seafood, vegetables, rice, and pickles, selected according to the season and presented with artistry. He will love the *bento* you prepare for your alfresco adventure to restore his weary soul in the bosom of nature. Whether you want to luxuriate in the scent of pine needles, new-mown grass, and swaying willow trees, or just listen to the roar of the ocean, you and your partner can enjoy a meal with that special sharpness and savor you'll only find outdoors. The preparation is already done. All you have to do is sit back and enjoy the romance of dining en plein air.

How to Make a Bento Box Tips

- A *bento* box is practical and quick. Do most of the cooking the night before: Cut the food into bite-size morsels so the only utensil he needs is your fingers.
- Start with the food that will take up the largest amount of space, such as rice, pasta, or sushi. You can use molds for shaping rice into manageable finger or chopstick size.
- Next, around the edges and stacked against the rice or pasta, add some green such as broccoli or asparagus, and then some red, such as tomato, to give the *bento* box appealing spots of bright color.
- Keep vinegary foods such as pickled ginger and salad apart from everything else, using cupcake liners, foil, or lettuce leaves.
- A plastic container with a tight-fitting lid is the best way to avoid spillage. Carry the box upright. Use wicker, wood, lacquer, or paper boxes.
- Don't forget the pretty, bright tablecloth with matching napkins, silverware or chopsticks, glasses, and other tableware.

diced shrimp artfully placed atop a tubular piece of white marble, learning the artful arrangement of food as well as its preparation is key to creating that sensual dinner for him. Invoke a new sensuality in your presentation, and you will inspire the romantic lure of the geisha serving him the finest cuisine with elegance and a sensual panache.

Cook your food with a Japanese inflection. Try a *panko*-crusted fried pork cutlet served with a dense sweet-and-sour sauce. *Panko* flakes are much lighter and crunchier than the ordinary breadcrumbs. Steaming bowls of noodles are hard to resist, swimming in a delicious elixir flecked with sweet fried onions and mushrooms sliced so thin they look like reflections in the tawny vegetable broth.

Be daring and a little messy. Whip up tempura and let him watch you whisk the batter, gossamer thin for vegetables, thicker for succulent shrimp. Then suggest he lick the spoon or whatever else his heart desires. Or have a naked fondue party and skinny dip yourself in your favorite sauce, one body part at a time. Play cool jazz in the background as you grill chicken, beef, and vegetables on your outdoor barbecue. Vegetables undergo a magical transformation on the grill, turning from mere vegetables into tempting treats. It's interactive eating that leads to interactive lovemaking.

Be inventive with what you serve. Include dishes that fuse a Japanese aesthetic with touches of chili, garlic, caviar, *and* you. Instead of gold flakes, sprinkle kisses upon his lips and tell him you are offering him *omakase,* a tasting menu. This philosophy is a very Japanese sentiment and requires him to leave the decisions up to you. He doesn't tell you what he wants, just when he wants you

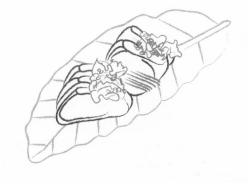

Sliced fresh fish for your menu: as sensual to look at as it is to offer your lover

to stop. It works in reverse as well. Just think—you don't have to ask him, you just tell him when (if ever!) to stop. Delish. He's hungry for dinner, then dessert: *you*. Don't disappoint him. Keep him under your spell by serving him a wonderful, delicious meal.

Sensual Food Tips

- *Salads*: Adjust the seasonings according to your taste—and his. He'll love the way the intriguing textures—crispy, crunchy, and crumbly—excite his taste buds.

- *Beef*: The merest whiff of beef sizzling on the grill drills straight through to the primitive part of his brain, making him hungry not just for steak but for you.

- *Fish*: For a special treat, prepare sweet shrimp with spicy lemon garlic sauce or shrimp tartare with truffles, caviar, and gold leaf on white daikon radish. Make sure your shrimp are perfect, tight skins on the outside with sweet, juicy flesh inside.

- *Desserts*: For a different taste treat, make a dessert with *yuzu*, one of the most popular citrus fruits in Japan. Its sweetly fragrant, slightly bitter zest is used to garnish dishes. You can use lemon or lime instead. Like you, citrus has complexity, a jazzy interplay of tart and sweet. Puddings can be sensuously rich, with the intensity of a dark chocolate truffle. Strawberry lime coolers are a refreshing and sensual delight. Use fresh strawberries, sugar, and the juice and zest of one lime. Purée strawberries, sugar, and lime juice until smooth, then serve over creamy ice cream.

- *Cap It Off*: You can sip a warm mug of fragrant green tea as a finale to a meal and a warm-up to the cozy activities you've planned for later on in the evening.

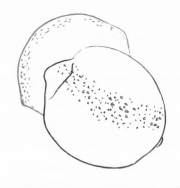

Citrus fruits like lemons and limes add
a jazzy interplay of tart and sweet

ALCOHOLIC SEDUCTION

Enjoying Western or Japanese wine, like making love, is an art, from looking at the liquid against a white background to judge the color, to swirling it in the glass to aerate it and send up a pungent burst of aroma, to taking the last sip. The scent should be pleasant. Swill or chew it about to give the wine a moment in your mouth as you evaluate its body. Body is a textural sensation. Focus on it. Savor the aftertaste, what is called the "finish." With a good wine—as with a night of good sex—the finish will pleasantly linger.

No meal served by a geisha or courtesan was complete without the drink of the gods: sake. Sake is an ancient elixir. First brewed in China nearly seven thousand years ago, it was introduced into Japan about two thousand years ago. There it became the delight of connoisseurs. In ancient times, beautiful young virgins made sake through a primitive process of chewing rice and spitting it into a large tub, thereby assuring its purity. The wine was aptly named *bijinshu,* "beauty wine."

But sake has always had a ribald, joyfully sensual side, as revealed in an *ukiyoe* print showing three men and three women sharing sake and delicacies amid the titillation of sexual exploits to come. Today customers at live sex clubs often hum along to the song *Sake Yo,* as they watch the action on stage and drink. Many drink so much at these raucous parties that sex is beyond their capabilities. They are, as geisha would say, more than *horoyoi,* "slightly intoxicated." You can sip sake while you're cooking a glorious meal

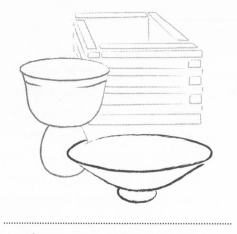

Sake cups come in a variety of shapes for cold, hot, and intimate imbibing

or watching the full moon, but be careful not to have too much of a good thing. Instead of him staying over, *you* will have a hangover.

With a crisp, clean taste and very subtle fruit, sake is excellent with sushi and harmonizes well with other dishes, including lightly prepared pasta, soy, vegetables, fish, and white meat. Sake is available in several grades. Premium sake is aged for six to nine months and should be consumed within one year of the bottling date. When you drink, you should drink well: The best sakes are as delicate—and as expensive—as fine wine.

It has been said the geisha could, as she poured sake into a tiny porcelain cup, make a gentleman feel as if he were the only man in the world. So can you with your lover. Here are some tips to help you.

SAKE TIPS

- Sake is delicious when heated. On a cold winter's night, it warms your hands and mouth, fires the spirit, and loosens inhibitions. *Yukimizake* is drinking sake while enjoying the snow—in an outdoor hot-spring or Jacuzzi with your man. Intense cold and heavy moist air make Japanese snow rich and frothy, like thick, ceremonial tea.

Samurai Rock: Fill a large glass one-third full of sake. Add ice and lime juice, stir, and drink.

Sake with Ice: Place sake in a glass with ice cubes and drink. Add a slice of lemon, if you wish. Lemon makes the taste milder.

Hot Sake: Place a container of sake in a pan of hot water and warm it to slightly more than your body heat. This is one of the best ways to drink sake, since at warm (but not hot) temperatures its qualities can be fully appreciated, especially if you're snuggled up with him on a cold night.

- Indulge in a sake party. Choose different kinds: *Daiginjo* is smoothest and lightest. Roughly filtered *nigori* appears cloudy. Infused sake contains fruit or other flavors.

- Regular sake, *futsushu*, often comes in a box and is the equivalent of box wine. This inexpensive brew is usually served heated. It is drinkable, but you wouldn't serve it to someone special.

- Sake contains no artificial preservatives. Once the bottle is opened, it is good for about one week in the refrigerator.

- Connoisseurs insist that the cold beverage be chilled to forty-five degrees Fahrenheit and served in a special, small glass. Sake that is traditionally warmed to a little over a hundred degrees and served in tiny ceramic cups is called *kan*[9] and is popular among some Japanese in the winter. It is up to you—and your man—which you prefer.

ICE

On a hot night, there is nothing sexier than a cool sliver of ice slithering down your nude body into the most interesting places. Keep cool. In the eleventh century, Heian ladies enjoyed ice preserved in chambers dug into the mountainsides. It was a summer luxury for members of the imperial court, including Sei Shonagon, who recorded her observations and personal reflections in lists like "Elegant Things," including "shaved ice mixed with liana syrup and put in a new silver bowl."[10]

Chilled foods are automatically sensual. Be creative with how you serve cold drinks to set a cool, sexy mood. Ice-frosted glass bowls and plates can hold everything from chilled fruit to sashimi and noodles. Serve sweets with frozen iced tea, or chilled water. Try serving shaved ice "Japanese style" by sweetening it with flavored syrups, condensed milk, or the green, thick tea of the tea ceremony (chilled before pouring) and topping it with sweet *azuki* beans. If this is not to your taste, try your own version of shaved ice with cups of crushed ice drenched with syrups that range from erotic tamarind and mango to kiwi-strawberry. Add a scoop of vanilla or chocolate ice cream between shaved ice balls on an oblong dish for a sweet and creamy treat.

AMBIANCE

A *kotatsu* is an irreplaceable cultural symbol in Japan. The low, quilt-covered table with a heat source below is about creating a cozy space as it is about physical warmth. At the *kotatsu*, formality gave way to physical intimacy and unrestrained familiarity. As the only warm spot in the wintertime teahouse, it was where geisha gathered for meals, talk, gossip, laughter, and exchanging stories about their lovers.[11]

Fireplaces are another welcome haven for you and your man to snuggle and make love. Place several soft, throw pillows or a furry rug on the floor; add a small low-to-the-floor table to hold drinks and snacks. Turn the lights low . . . and the rest is up to you.

You can create a romantic, sensual scene with the right kind of magic. It's all in the details, from charming napkin holders and fresh flowers, to overhead lights shielded with amber glass shades, to discreet wood paneling, to wide-body comfortable chairs big enough for two to snuggle. Or be glamorous for your favorite night owl by hanging Chinese lanterns over a small outdoor bar and letting them sway in the breeze. Sit on a high bar stool in your backless dress, surrounded by flickering votive candles. Do a funky "come-as-you-are" brasserie setting and serve upmarket comfort food. Buy a couple of shaggy ottomans, add some plants, and string piazza lights in strategic places. The soft, casual atmosphere makes it a favorite escape and enhances the sense of cozy privacy. Get all lovey-dovey on your comfy outdoor swing draped with a canopy of golden silk and lit by ornate Moroccan lanterns. Scatter your pool with rose petals before taking that midnight skinny dip, and set up lounge chairs with fluffy robes waiting, along with shaken cocktails or espresso martinis. Get crazy. Howl at the moon. In between, nibble on homemade potato chips, fried olives, cheeses—and each other.

A FINAL NOTE ON SETTING THE MOOD FOR SEDUCTION . . .

Setting the mood for seduction is similar to the classical art of Noh theater. After the dance had been carefully choreographed, the dancer could then allow his performance to develop of itself. If you want to allow the evening to develop freely into a night of romance and lovemaking, check on everything that *shouldn't* be noticed: the temperature of the room, the scents, the lighting, and the soundtrack. The less obvious the effect, the better. You want to bring him into an environment that overcomes physical and emotional stress and out-side distractions, that nurtures and inspires as it pleasures and relaxes you both. Make your home friendly, and seduction will surely follow.

Chapter 5

IKI: THE ART OF COOL

The geisha of Tatsumi goes walking,
Bare white feet in black lacquered clogs.
In her haori jacket, she's the pride of Great Edo.
Ah, the Hachiman Bell is ringing.

Anonymous *ko-uta*, geisha song[1]

Imagine a beautiful geisha, tall and graceful, bright red toenails accenting her bare white feet, standing amid a crowd of merrymakers on a verandah near a snowdrift. Delicately, she points her toes toward the snow. The conversation stops; everyone turns to watch her. They hold their breath. Undaunted, she smiles, then walks boldly into the cold drifts. *That*, to the Japanese of Old Edo, was the height of *iki*, an erotic sense of style and polish exemplified by certain geisha and courtesans. We call it "cool."

Although the act of walking through the snow in itself dramatized *iki*, it was the quality of character implied by the act that made her truly *iki*.[2] That quality was wildly erotic to artists of the Edo period, who defined the epitome of the *iki* aesthetic in woodblock prints of kimono-clad geisha depicted with long, clean lines and subtle, subdued hues.[3] Being *iki* was about having an impact. You can achieve that same impact when you enter a room, meet someone for the first time, flirt. It's a quality men can't resist.

So, how do you get it? First, let's define *iki*.

Iki was "cool," "chic." It had an element of daring and unconventionality, yet was the opposite of contrived. Its aim was a simple, striking elegance of inner character that manifested itself in outer dress and manner. It fed on the masculine ego and libido. It invoked an understated sensuality that was only hinted at, never flaunted. *Iki* geisha and courtesans never wore *tabi*, the dainty white socks of ordinary women; the *haori*, a man's loose jacket, sported over their kimono added a vague intimation of associations with the opposite sex. *That* was flair.

THE THREE ELEMENTS OF *IKI*

- The first element is *hari*, spirit: a sharp, direct, and uncompromising social style both balanced and cool, as well as bravely composed. This is what you develop when you practice *kokono-tokoro* to perfection.

- The second element is *bitai*, coquetry or allure: flirtatiousness with restrained eroticism. A woman who possesses *bitai* is charming but not vulgar or wanton.

- The third element is *akanuke*, urbanity, stylishness, or polish that is unassuming and unpretentious. An aspect of disinterest that suggests the ideal beauty is restrained, not necessarily perfect, and always pleasant.

Iki originated in the Asakusa district of the capital city of Edo in the seventeenth century. It was a time when the Tokugawa shoguns had closed the country's doors to foreigners, leaving the populace to look inward for its pleasures. Asakusa was the cultural mecca for the decadent pop culture of *ukiyo*, "the floating world." It was a place of sake shops and teahouses, streets crowded with acrobats, jugglers, musicians, and vendors selling everything from toys and sweets to erotic woodblock prints. The carnival-like atmosphere revolved around the twin poles of the nearby Yoshiwara licensed brothel quarters, crowded with beautiful, expensive women, and the flamboyant Kabuki theater with its aerial stunts, brilliant staging and costuming, and acting bravado.

Asakusa raised its "cool quotient" higher during the Meiji period (1868–1912), when Japan's first photography studios opened there. The first skyscraper, first movie theater, and first cabarets and music halls were located there, as well as Japan's first bar, which opened in 1880 and still exists. Tokyo's "cool" districts today include the Ginza and Akasaka, where you can find hostess clubs catering to a masculine clientele seeking a sensual place of relaxation and comfort. These clubs do not provide sex, but are purveyors of the traditional stylishness of *iki* for the businessmen, bankers, and politicians who run Japan.

Is your town *iki*? Wherever you live, cool rules. You just have to look for it. From NYC to LA, from Chicago to New Orleans and everywhere in between, look around you. We have our own cool culture and it's different everywhere you go. Frequent the kinds of places that reflect your idea of "cool" and the men you want to attract will find *you*.

IKI AND SEX APPEAL

A geisha or courtesan with *iki* wore a subdued kimono, but her pose hinted at the certain coquettishness that sparkled beneath. She displayed sexual charm by her discreetly exposed chest, the nape of her neck, and as she walked, the flash of her leg against her red underslip,[4] all risqué at the time. The grace of her left hand holding her robes closed contributed to her fascination, as did her triple-width petticoat, tied rather higher than women not of her profession.[5] For the man who gazed at her, she personified the realm of potential conquest. Her experience and intensity, her previous illicit relationships, all evident from her dress, walk,

"Iki-cetera"

What is *iki* is as changeable as the seasons. One thing is for sure: If you don't like what's in, wait around awhile. It will go out. Here are some "*iki*-cetera" items that have the "cool" factor:

- *Parasols*: Japanese have used umbrellas for a thousand years; some are considered works of art. The earliest, covered with silk and not closable, were status symbols. Because beautiful skin was important to the geisha and courtesan's art of seduction, they protected themselves with parasols whenever they went outdoors. *Ukiyoe* often depict sumptuously dressed young women holding them. Geisha used a *karakasa*, made from oiled-paper, silk, and bamboo, brightly colored, and lightweight. A special lacquer made it water-repellent, and an aromatic oil gave it a distinctive scent. Even today, Kabuki actors use them to enhance the grace and flow of their dances. You can be *iki* and summer cool with a parasol. Get a little sun umbrella. Unlike a hat, it won't ruin your hair and it is *so* sexy.

- *Beautiful Underwear* is always *iki*. It is elegant, but hidden. You can't help but feel sexy.

- *Shopping Bags*, as integral to Japanese culture as the tea ceremony, have risen from the simply utilitarian to a moving advertisement of "cool"—an essential fashion accessory as well as a status symbol. If the shopping bag is nice, it is believed the quality of the merchandise inside is also nice, as in what you wear outside reflects the sexy you underneath. If you shop in a discount store, put your purchases in an expensive-looking shopping bag.

and demeanor, only inflamed his desire for what he himself had yet to attain—and might never. *Iki* developed from all these ambient factors into a cultural phenomenon of style, mood, and harmony.

When a woman with *iki* discovered she was the object of a man's passionate obsession, the next move was up to her. She made inquiries, discreetly, of course, to discover if he had the knowledge and style to play her seductive game. She was quick to assess if he qualified as an expert or connoisseur. After all, her reputation was at stake. To prove worthy, he must also possess a sensitivity to her heart, this woman of his desire, as well as knowledge of the rules on which the world of pleasure she inhabited was built. Finally, she looked for a man with the self-discipline to play his role in a way that sustained the magic.

Next, you will explore these factors in depth and learn how *iki* can help *you* seduce him. Although the nature of socializing and sexuality has changed since these times, the basic elements of *iki* have not. Erotic allure not being easily attainable, possessing a certain style will attract men to you.

LOOKING *IKI*

The *iki* way of dressing came about with a shift from elaborately luxurious kimono toward a more muted approach to dress. And, because of its association with geisha and high-ranking courtesans, always arbiters of fashion, a deep eroticism underlay this look and contributed to its fascination. *Iki* was refinement, an aesthetic philosophy based on a sense of beauty where understated outward display hinted at deep feeling within. A stray hair, a glimpse of red at the collar of a gray striped kimono, a quiet sophistication and restrained chic in both appearance *and* behavior. Such a woman had tasted the bitterness of life as well as the sweet, and appreciated both. *That* made her *iki*.

But *iki* was not conservative or dull. Something also could be *iki* because it was original—unconventional without being overt. That is why a geisha defined *iki* as "always being prepared." She would spend hours bathing, dressing, doing her makeup and her hair, even if she had "nowhere to go." It was a lesson in discipline, manners, and observation around the single theme of being ready for whatever might happen. You can use this same strategy in setting your own personal style. Don't wait until that special night to try out a new hairdo or makeup or outfit. Learn ahead of time what colors look best, what fabrics and styles flatter, what your best features are, how to minimize your less attractive ones,

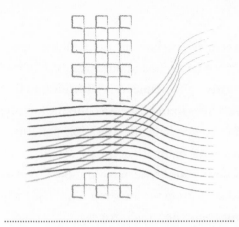

Typical iki textile patterns were often simple stripes and checks in plain colors

and how to mix and match basic pieces with accessories.

The basic shape of the kimono never changed, but it conveyed much of the wearer's financial status, family background, and personality. The geisha's was a one-of-a-kind work of art, reflecting her personal style. Your clothes likewise reflect your personality. Learn how to identify quality. Look for markdowns if you can't afford haute couture. Think "elegant" and "classy," and it will show. And, follow that basic rule of *iki* elegance: Less is better than more. Too many accessories can cheapen your look. Be simple, but be striking.

When the Heian lady wished to inflame a suitor's desires, she would simply let him catch a glimpse of her multi-layered sleeve through her carriage window or curtain. This was enough to send even the most stoic gentleman into romantic frenzy. A thousand years later, *iki* geisha and courtesans used their beautiful, subtle sense of style in dress to attract men, intimating artistic sophistication or sexual innuendo in an extremely wide sash without any inner lining, *ohabaobi*,[6] loosely tied with a dangling knot. It is not just the style of clothing you choose, but also the fabric, cut, and how it hugs your body.

IKI COLOR

Iki can be defined as a harmony of the whole and a harmony of detail. It is exemplified by the landscape of Japan, which is filled with discreet, blending hues: fields of golden rape-seed and bamboo forests of deep green; delicate violet wisterias and pure white camellias; dark brown, old wooden farmhouses and white castle walls; maple trees with autumn leaves like tongues of red fire. These sensual yet restrained hues found their way into the kimono of geisha of taste. Many *ukiyoe* depict these elegant women in textiles of simple patterns, reflecting the peaceful yet sophisticated aspect that is the hallmark of the *iki* style.

Color is extremely important in determining your style. Here are some ways to consider a few basic, essential colors to help you decide upon the look you want. Use them as a model for thinking of other colors, and the messages they might convey:

- *Blue*: Cool, serene color of the water and sky. Deep blue is chic, like black. Softer blues are restful and soothing.

- *Green*: Deep or soft greens take from both the liveliness of yellow and the calm effect of the blue. Wear green when you want to keep him guessing about your mood.

- *Violet*: Light pastel violet suggests a feminine yet slightly eccentric style. Wear this color when you want to be coy and flirtatious. Deep, rich violet or purple transmit a warm dignity and splendor, perfect for the night you want to be queenly.

An *iki* woman knew that strong colors should be used sparingly—this is when they have the most impact. In small amounts, intense color is a subtle hint of a smoldering nature, one that is passionate, playful, and sparkling only when the time is right. Use strong colors as accents: small streaks and patches of bright in elegantly neutral prints; a striking blouse or sweater beneath a chic, dark jacket; a bright piece of beautiful jewelry peaking from beneath a cuff or through your hair:

- *Red*: The color of fire; it imparts a feeling of warmth and excitement.

- *Yellow*: Suggests warm sunshine and is light and cheerful. Wear yellow when you want your personality to sparkle and shine.

- *Orange*: Mixed from red and yellow, orange is both cheerful and exciting, but not as vibrant as its primary cousins. Orange can make you feel succulent and playful.

CLOTHING TIPS

- The courtesan wore a long robe whose sleeves measured two feet and five inches. Draw the eye by wearing a piece of clothing that catches the wind, like a long, chiffon scarf or billowy full sleeves, or a hanging belt a lover can grab as you walk by.

- She also wore an exceptionally wide *obi*, with the knot tied higher than usual. Try wearing a tight bustier or corset-like piece over a loose dress or blouse and pants. A tight, nipped-in waist is very sexy and makes you sway your hips more as you walk. It will also help you keep in your stomach and make your breasts look bigger.

- The *maiko* enchanted the eye and ear with her long, long *obi* trailing down her back and six-inch-high wooden sandals, *okobo*, fastened with tiny bells. Develop your own head-turning outfit with understated glamour and mystique. Keep accessories to a minimum, but striking.

- Reach for your favorite basic little black dress and sexy high heels when you want instant polish and easy elegance. Carry it off with impeccable posture.

- The colors and patterns of the kimono are endless and change with the season as well as the age of the wearer. Be careful about the message you send by wearing clothing that is appropriate to the occasion and your age.

IKI COMMUNICATION

The word *geisha* is derived from two characters: *gei*, meaning "art," and *sha*, meaning "person." It is not coincidence that "art" came first, since it was the most important thing in the geisha's life. In addition to dancing and singing, she learned to play many musical instruments, including the *tsutsumi*, hand drum. Geisha were also skilled in the fine arts of calligraphy and poetry. You can develop *iki*-essence by cultivating an art. Break out of your traditional role, be expressive, and open up by empowering yourself, especially in the art of communication.

When geisha entered an *ozashiki*, *maiko* entered first, while the oldest—and most revered—geisha entered last. The pretty young *maiko* giggled as they poured the sake, but the older geisha, with her witty conversation, extensive knowledge, and ability to make the customer feel sexy and important, sparkled the brightest. Where did she get this goddess-like sexuality with words? It was part of her—and your—genetic makeup. You are smart. Your conversation will also sparkle irresistibly if you follow these tips.

EROTIC CONVERSATION TIPS

- When you compliment your lover, avoid scripted dialogue that sounds like you read it in a novel or heard it in a film, or if you've said the same thing to other men. Find something unique. If he's worth your time, the words will come naturally.

- In days gone by, geisha teahouses were often the sites of political intrigues. One of the geisha's most endearing traits was her ability to keep a secret. Don't tell your girlfriends every detail of your last lovemaking session. If your lover knows you to be discreet about your private moments, he will be back for more.

- Geisha knew how important it was to let men talk about what interests them. Men love to be asked for their views about a subject, so bring up current events and discuss them. Don't be afraid to challenge him with your own opinions. Men love to argue—and no one loses when you end up in bed together.

- Just as a Heian lady's beauty and charm were measured by her skill in coordinating the kaleidoscopic layers of her silk kimono, you will be captivating as a woman who is forever revealing another interesting layer of personality. Having a medley of interests can add dimension to your relationship because you are bringing more intrigue to the table, and more raw material to discuss.

- In the golden days of Yoshiwara, the *tayu* chose her clients—or rejected those not to her liking. This kept a man waiting with bated breath, never knowing if she was going to sleep with him. The pleasure centers of your lover's brain are most strongly activated by the unanticipated. Throw him an occasional curveball to keep your relationship fresh.

- The geisha or *geiko* of Kyoto had their own delicious dialect that turned on any man. You *can* talk dirty to your man, but test the waters first to find his comfort level. Some men find "naughty talk" a turn-on; others don't.

EROTIC LOVE LETTERS

> My letter written in common character will be worth more than a verbal message.[7]

After making love, the eighteenth-century heroine Osuki composed a letter to the current gentleman of her bedchamber; with it she placed three of her pubic hairs as a sign of her affection.[8] Sei Shonagon, the Heian-era author of *The Pillow Book,* expressed her feelings in a different manner. She used a witty anecdote, knowing that bringing a smile to the face heightens the eroticism of love letters. Each lady wrote with rich literary allusion, in skillful calligraphy. Each chose just the right *washi*, handmade paper, upon which to compose, attached a delicate blossom or autumn sprig to evoke the correct sentiments and season, and scented the paper with the perfect fragrance. Send your lover a handwritten love note. It's easy, effective, rich with expressive possibilities, and full of delight for both of you. Don't forget to seal the envelope with a lipstick kiss in his favorite color. Try getting *that* into an email.

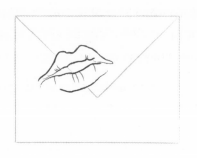

Seal your intimate love letter with a tasteful lipstick kiss

Love letters are the written history of a romance, allowing lovers to rediscover what they feel about each other. They prolong the magic in a relationship by connecting each to those specific shared moments. With the prevalence of modern electronic communication, as long lasting as a sigh, a real, erotic love letter is truly *iki*. Below are some tips to help you compose your own. Whether or not you add any "personal" touches inside your envelope, as Osuki did, is up to you.

WRITING LOVE LETTERS BY HAND

In a classic scene from *The Tale of Genji*, Lady Murasaki dismisses a younger, more beautiful rival for her husband's attention once she sees the lady's immature calligraphy. How is *your* handwriting? Neat and easily read? Or, a jumble of undotted i's and uncrossed t's? Practice with a calligraphy pen. This old-fashioned object can be a link to your heart.

Handwriting is an intensely personal form of communication. When a lover receives your handwritten letter, he knows you took time especially for him, that there are only the two of you, and that you speak differently when writing than in person or on the phone. A handwritten letter shows him that you care. You are conveying how you feel to him, and if you feel sexy, that's more likely to show in your handwriting. It reveals another layer in your personality that makes you all the more intriguing.

IMPROVE YOUR HANDWRITING TIPS

- Handwriting is a basic part of your everyday life so it only makes sense to make it part of your sex life as well. Just as most women don't have perfect bodies, most women—and men—don't have perfect handwriting. Don't worry. It's those imperfections that make your handwriting so special to him.

- Make writing a pleasure. Do it while listening to romantic music in a pleasant spot. Buy a special pen to use only for love letters, like the elegant Namiki fountain pen, the choice of tasteful Japanese women since 1925. Made with *makie*, sprinkled gold powder on lacquer, Namiki pens are exquisitely decorated in layered patterns on the barrel and cap. All these elements make writing its own reward, not to mention the extra special loving you will get later from him.

Writing Erotic Love Letters Tips

- A love letter is like chocolate. When it is good, it is *really* good. And when it's bad, it's still pretty good. Don't try to be perfect. It will make your writing sound awkward or superficial.

- An email can't carry a hint of your perfume or be saved in his desk drawer. Besides, you never know who is reading *his*. If you must send an email love note, be creative but not trendy with your words. "I luv U 4-ever" may brighten his day, but lacks your personal touch.

- Try making your own pretty *shikishi*, rectangular or fan-shaped writing papers, like those in use since the eighth century to mark special occasions. Traditionally, a *shikishi* is inscribed with a poem in beautiful calligraphy. Decorate your *shikishi* with little photos of you, poems you wrote, and cutouts of things special to both of you to convey your dreams, hopes, and sexy thoughts.

- Don't write, "I think you're really hot," or the names you have picked out for your children, or use the L-word. Don't say you love him unless you mean it.

- Write about the special times you have spent together: How you feel when he makes love to you, the emotions that run through you when your hands are touching, your lips locking. Avoid discussing body parts, his or yours, and keep it a love letter.

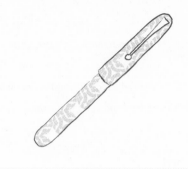

Write love letters with a Namiki fountain pen,
the choice of tasteful Japanese women for decades

LEAVING AN ELEGANT IMPRESSION

When a *maiko* called on important persons or delivered a geisha's thank-you note for a gift, she left behind her oblong *meishi*. This charming card was inscribed with her name and address in flowing calligraphy, and an exquisite design often in black or red lacquer outlined with a gold. The beautiful little cards were coveted by admirers as special mementos of affection. You can be memorable in the same way. Use a scanner and your personal printer to make your own *meishi* with your signature and a design.

If you want to be truly unforgettable, use a letterpress card to which you have added a *hanko*, name stamp. A *hanko* is a small cylinder carved on one end with characters that, when stamped in ink, leave the owner's imprint. It is a custom with deep cultural roots. Japan's first evidence of the written word was a solid-gold *hanko* dating to A.D. 57. *Hanko* initially were used only by the emperor as an extension of his authority. Nobles adopted them in Heian times. Samurai followed in the Edo period, claiming an exclusive right to use red ink. The general public took up the custom after 1868.

Most Japanese have several *hanko*. Men's are generally bigger than women's.

Yugen and Sexy Body Language

Yugen means "quiet beauty," "elegant simplicity," "subtle," and "profound." The occult is *yugen*. "*Yugen* may be comprehended by the mind, but it cannot be expressed in words. Its quality may be suggested by the sight of a thin cloud veiling the moon or by autumn mist swathing the scarlet leaves on a mountainside."[a]

Because *yugen* is the mark of supreme attainment in all the arts and accomplishments, the highest achievement in beauty of form and manner, perhaps it is the best word to describe a geisha's grace, from her walk to her dance to the tilt of her head. To truly understand *yugen*, never forget that the effect of the geisha's physical presence grows from the balance she achieves between her mental and physical actions.

Yugen also favors intimation over plain statement—as with the geisha in her art of seduction: what she expressed with her body and what she knew, but did not overtly say. When slowly raising her hands in dance, it might have been only part of her performance, but yet again could have been to one man the message of a gateway to a night of lovemaking.

As you acquire mastery of your movements, you will come to understand beyond what you have learned. What you *suggest* with your body rather than *express* is the true art of seduction.

Hanko can be made from anything hard enough to make an imprint: wood, crystal, shell, plastic, ivory, jade, agate, titanium, gold, buffalo horn, and even woolly mammoth fossils. They can cost as much as $20,000 for a 24-karat gold and ivory stamp nestled in a crocodile-skin case, and as little as eighty cents for something of molded plastic.

Run your fingers across a letterpress card and you can feel the subtle landscape created by inked metal pressed into the paper. Stores selling fine papers often sell a selection of stamps. You can choose something with an initial or a symbol that says "you," or have one made to order. If you want to be *really iki*, carve one yourself.

IKI BODY ART: TATTOOS

The geisha wore the collar of her kimono low in the back so her bare skin could be seen.

This made a man more aware of the living, breathing woman under her alabaster mask. If he was her lover, he might have known that hidden somewhere beneath those perfumed, silken robes, his name adorned her naked skin. This was a testament of their intimacy and her passion. Done right, tattoos can be *iki*.

Tattooists call themselves *horishi*, from the verb *horu*, "to dig or carve." The tattoo is called *horimono*, which sounds elegant, like engraving. An *iki* courtesan or geisha was as restrained about her tattoo as she was about her kimono. Nothing loud, large, or colorful for her. Her tattoo was simple and chic, even a little severe. The most common were the *kanji*, characters, of her lover's name. The visual force of Japanese characters is dramatic and powerful, and has its own beauty.

Tattoos used to be taboo in our culture, but not anymore. Ten percent of Americans have a tattoo. They can be sexy and fun, a way to incorporate a special experience such as a significant birthday, job promotion, divorce, or engagement. They can suggest the exotic, the "forbidden fruit." They can be your testament as a woman with a more interesting and broader view of the world, especially when you choose a *kanji*. The most commonly requested are those for "beauty," "love," "woman," "strength," and "happiness."

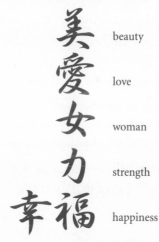

美 beauty

愛 love

女 woman

力 strength

幸福 happiness

Some popular characters for tattoos that can tastefully convey your outlook on life

TATTOO TIPS

- Tattooing hurts more on areas with little padding, like your spine, wrists, and ankles.

- Many tattoo artists are women, making the experience more comfortable if you decide you want your genitalia adorned with a tattoo.

- Some dangers are involved, like a skin reaction to the dyes used and the spread of infectious diseases. Latex gloves and autoclave sterilizers are now commonplace. Make sure your tattoo artist uses them.

- You can always opt for the temporary rub-on tattoos if you don't want a permanent one. Use a marker or ballpoint pen to make a sketch on your breasts or legs. You can keep the tattoo on for a couple of days before washing it off.

"*IKI*-MODERN": BODY PIERCINGS

Although she never wore earrings or belly rings, a courtesan recognized the sensual attraction of shiny objects in dazzling her customer. She coifed her black hair in elaborate coils and loops adorned with sparkling silver hairpins, *kanzashi*, and her sash clasp, *potchiri*, worn near her belly button, was often studded with a diamond. But a courtesan who was *iki* had "an edge." Today, that means body piercings.

PIERCING TIPS

- Your belly, *hara*, is *iki* and from it you derive your breath and strength.[9] Your belly is also the center of your true feelings and emotions. Why not adorn it with your own personal diamond stud or belly ring?

- Body piercings have their practical side. A button in your tongue allows you to give your man a myriad of wild sensations during oral sex.

While unthinkable in Old Japan, body piercings today represent a modern form of chic

- Don't rule out genital piercings. A piercing in your clitoral hood adds erotic sensation to manual or oral sex. A piercing in the head of his penis can give you the illusion of deeper penetration, and a ladder (a series of barbell piercings along the underside of his penis) adds stimulation to your vaginal walls during intercourse.

IKI-ESSENCE

Iki fuses emotions with aesthetic ideals. That's a philosophy for "cool," no matter what kind. *Iki* is having what the Japanese call the "inner core of experience," a certain nonchalance toward the ups and downs of life—and men. No matter what she was feeling inside, if her heart was broken or her mood sad, when a geisha entered a banquet, she sought out the person in the place of honor and engaged him in a charming conversation as if he were the most important person in her life. In that moment, she was truly *iki*. She was, as the Japanese say, "looking at the rocks and sand with the eyes of the heart."[10]

Don't show your feelings if things aren't going your way or if you are rejected.

Don't be led against your wishes. Don't act insecure, try to keep him on a leash, or change a lover. This rarely, if ever, succeeds. A woman with *iki* would never involve herself with a man who needs changing. What he is as man, gentleman and lover, she finds desirable at the outset, hence her interest in him. She is spontaneous, less demanding, and independent minded; in other words, seeming *disinterest* makes *her* interesting. As a woman with *iki*, you will find you have the upper hand. He, of course, won't know.

When she saw a flower, in declaring it beautiful the *iki* woman experienced not merely its physical presence, but also its freshness and brightness. Look beyond appearances and seek the essence of everyone and everything. Be aware of how a change in the wind blows the silk of your scarf against your face and cools the blush of your cheek, or how the light filtering through a window casts a different glow on a hardwood floor, giving it a mystical quality, an *iki* quality. Like the geisha, whose highest accolade was to be gossiped about as being *iki*, you can acquire this in many different—and unusual—ways. It adds up to a rarefied elegance and interest so that something about you transcends the ordinary.

Your look, style, and attitude tell a story about you. They make the difference between whether you plod along or sashay with an erotic tease in your step. You can create a graceful harmony by considering your hairdo, your jewelry, your suit jacket, and even your lingerie according to a unified philosophy of taste. And, when these shapes,

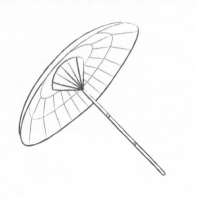

For a woman who wants to make an impression, a parasol is a useful fashion accessory

colors, patterns, scents, and sounds are in concordance, you feel better about yourself and exude self-confidence because you know *you* are at your best. You will have charisma.

Iki is a natural part of your femininity. You have but to bring it out. As a character of the famed erotic novelist Ihara Saikaku said, "I had not yet blossomed, yet as far as love was concerned, I had already experienced sensual pleasure just as the blossom of a Yamabuki yellow rose already possesses the proper color before it opens."[11]

You are like the yellow rose, waiting to open for the right man.

Chapter 6

THE ART OF PLAY

Low words followed by high laughter:
It must be something really funny!

Anonymous *senryu* (Edo-period satirical verse)[1]

The two young geisha, arms full of pompoms made of fresh chrysanthemums, winked at each other as they began their game of tossing a shower of blooms at each other. They knew they were being watched! The many-colored chrysanthemum balls flew through the air, long ribbons streaming like white and red meteors; their bittersweet perfume mingled with incense burning in the alcove, filling the room.[2] When the gentleman made his presence known, the taller girl giggled, then tossed a ball of flowers and hit him on the back. This was playtime, geisha style.

When a geisha playfully threw a light object at a man—a ball of paper, a match, etc., this was a coquettish gesture indicating she was interested in him.[3] She could also expect to be on the receiving end of flamboyantly playful games from her admirers. The famed O-Koi once found herself at an evening's entertainment with several distinguished businessmen dressed up like students in navy-blue outfits, drinking from casks of sake. The men ran after her all night, breaking furniture and trying to get her out of her kimono.[4] Such games were commonplace in the life of a geisha.

Play is any activity you do because it feels good. Sexy and provocative, it is an important element in your art of seduction. You can be funny, flirtatious, flattering, and funky in a physical manner. Play loosens inhibitions. Don't underestimate its power to increase the depth of your relationship. All play is sexy. Not all play has to end in intercourse. That is what makes it "play." Knowing this takes the pressure off both of you. You and your lover deserve time for it.

HUMOR TIPS

- Geisha were wonderful at making their guests laugh. Don't forget to laugh, especially at yourself. Look for the humor in the things around you. Let your hair down more often. Do something silly and spontaneous.

- Humor can be found in almost any situation. It is individual, as well as mutual. Sometimes you will see the humor in something; other times, both of you will share a humorous moment.

- Humor diffuses an awkward situation: on a first date, or when your bra strap breaks or that "sale" tag is hanging out of the back of your dress (giving you an excuse to invite him to tuck the tag inside and run his fingers over your bare skin). You can't always choose what is going to happen, but you *can* control how you react to it.

- Remember: Many times, you can't laugh at something when it is happening; but in the end, it can be your best "date from hell" story. And, stories are to share. . . .

- Letting go of stress may be as easy as laughing.

Fans

In the late nineteenth century, a popular geisha in the Tokyo Shinbashi district carried a fan that opened wide to display an ink-drawn picture depicting a famous Japanese tale—Rashomon and the dragon. To entertain her customer, the geisha flipped the fan partly closed. As she did so, the drawings transformed

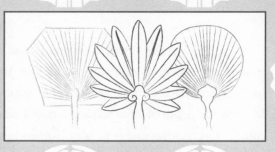

themselves into anatomically correct images of the male and female genitalia. Folding the fan again, she completed the act of making love.[a]

The Empress Jingo Kogo invented the folding fan, called *ogi* in the third century. *Uchiwa* are flat fans with handles. Every Heian lady, geisha, and courtesan carried one or the other. When a geisha danced, she carried a *maiogi*, a fan with bamboo spines about twelve inches long. There were many other kinds, for both men and women.

A fan was not merely a dainty feminine trifle; it was the flirt's secret weapon. She held hers differently from a man, using body language to make it sexually titillating. Sliding her legs to the side, she would arch her neck slightly, and hold it with her thumb on the inside, moving her hand and wrist languorously. Resting the fan on her left cheek meant she was not interested. On the right, it meant "come hither." Drawn across her eyes meant "I am sorry." Drawn across her cheek meant "I love you." Putting the handle to her lips was an invitation to kiss—where things went from there, no fan was needed.[b] Even today, fans are the regulation gift upon every occasion. At feasts each guest receives a plain white *ogi*, upon which to write poems and sign autographs. You can entertain your lover by writing naughty poems on his fan. Later, when you are alone, it is a wonderful way of remembering the heat between the two of you, although it is doubtful this little summer fan will cool you off.

FLIRTING

At dusk, a courtesan would arrive at an *ageya*, trysting house, and enter with a rustling of silk and a fluttering of *tamoto*, the long, wing-like sleeves of her kimono. Smiling with a delicate nod to her waiting guest, she would go to sit beside him, taking his hand as she talked to him, admiring his clothing, his fan, her deft touch intimate yet restrained. She would closely watch the little porcelain sake cups, never allowing them to be empty or remain full. Each movement was flirtatious and carefully calculated to put the guest in a good mood and make him feel as if he was on the brink of paradise. Even the most insensitive of men could not resist this display of coquettishness. You can put your man in a paradise-like state if you follow these simple flirting techniques.

Flirting Tips

- The famous O-Koi knew how to captivate her guests: She left at ten o'clock, an early hour for a geisha party, so she would always be missed. Shoo him out of your place before he is ready to go. Don't worry. He'll be back.

- Don't be shy about flirting with your date. The courtesan was an expert. She would titillate by pretending to be reluctant, showing affection without undoing her *obi*, or lying down without displaying any eagerness. Men love the attention and the sense of challenge. He'll be running after you long after the date is over.

- Playing the innocent virgin can be a turn-on to some men. Try it with your lover. Losing your virginity a second time can be fun.

- In almost all geisha houses it is common to have a good-luck shelf facing the street full of *maneki neko*, "beckoning cats," each with a little paw raised enticingly. Don't be shy about sexy body movement. As you undress, slide one bra strap down your shoulder and give him that "come hither" look that lets him know what you are doing is especially for him.

- When a geisha really liked a man, she invited him to sit on her right. Why? She knew that side to be more alluring. Kimono were always worn with the left side crossed over the right. This made it easy for her to bestow a special favor to a deserving admirer—the chance to slip in his hand and fondle her breasts. Keep this in mind when you wear that sexy, new sweater with the buttons undone.

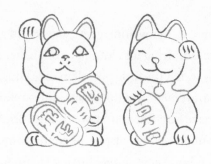

Beckoning cats are a friendly and light-hearted way of extending your welcome

- Be involved in what is going on with your man instead of worrying about how you look or what you said. The heart of any date is what's happening between the two of you. Taking a chance exploring the unknown often yields unexpectedly wonderful results.

- A *tayu* enjoyed the privilege of turning away a guest who did not please her. You have the same option on any date.

- What if flirting is the *last* thing on your mind with a man? The courtesan communicated lack of desire in fascinating ways: A knot tied in the sash of her *nagajuban*, underslip, would send an unmistakable message. If a man on whom she had bestowed her favors did not satisfy her, she would place hot ashes under

Old-Fashioned Geisha Games

- An eggplant and a pumpkin quarreling. The geisha blows out her cheeks like a pumpkin and the man falls down on top of her.
- The baseball game. The *maiko* pretends to throw the ball and the man pretends to hit it—and grabs her beautiful derrière.
- *Janken-pon*: "Scissors cut paper, paper wraps stone, stone breaks scissors." Thrust the hand forward with two fingers extended, or palm flat, or fist clenched. In the sexy version, the geisha had to spread her legs every time she lost, opening her kimono a little wider each time.
- Bumpsy daisy: The man stands on a cushion, back to back with a geisha. At the count of three, they bump their behinds together so the geisha loses balance and falls—and the gentleman catches her.
- This erotic game is quite a trick: The gentleman, balancing an apple sitting on a plate on top of his head, sits astride a geisha lying on her back. He bends forward and tries to take in his teeth a piece of paper the geisha holds in her mouth. This is a "touchy-feely" game where the man often ends up with more than paper in his mouth.
- A card game called *hanafuda*, introduced by Dutch sailors at the end of sixteenth century. There are forty-eight cards, each decorated with a flower design. The "forty-eight ways," *shiju-hachi te*, of sexual positions are based on the ways a sumo wrestler can defeat his opponent. The rules of the game are like sex: whatever is agreeable to the players.

the bedclothes near his feet to awaken him from deep sleep, then oust him from her bedchamber. Don't be afraid to show a lack of interest, but be subtle rather than crass in sending the message.

BECOME A CFO: FLATTER HIM

Yoshida Hanbei, in a 1686 work entitled *An Illustrated Manual of Eroticism*, describes how to tell if you are a sensuous woman:

You read love stories, you begin to seek adventures without thinking about eating. You can become lost in a whirlpool of pleasure without noticing that the night is ending or that the sun is rising. Moreover, whenever you encounter a man you cough audibly and you gaze lovingly at him.[5]

That means *flatter* him. Quick wit, excellent timing, a bit of irony, and a ton of praise can turn you into a CFO: Chief Flattery Officer. Clever conversation, storytelling skills, and the ability to improvise help prevent social mishaps. Subtle compliments give a positive glow to the atmosphere. This type of flattery is known as *yoisho*, "heavy lifting."[6] For example, a courtesan might speak highly of her guest's son, knowing that it would reflect positively on the guest. *Yoisho* is something to keep in mind when trying to impress *your* date, especially in the company of others. You can improve the mood by indulging him in a pick-him-up minute of ego boosting to make certain he is feeling good about himself. And if you can't do it in person, there's always the telephone. *Hello*, phone sex, anyone?

EROTIC PHONE SEX TIPS

- Whether your lover lives in the same city or across the country, phone sex is fun sex. According to a survey conducted by a woman's magazine, eighty-five percent of men want women to make that breathy call.[7] So, see what happens when you say more than "*hello*."

- On the phone you can test the limits and say those sexy things you might be too intimidated to tell him in person.

- Ask questions to get your lover thinking about being with you intimately. Does

- Change your bedroom light bulb for one tinted red and invite your lover over for a fiery surprise. The ruby rays kick-start an erotic response in the both of you. The red highlights on your lips, cheeks, and breasts make you look flushed as if sexually excited and instantly more appealing. Red light is proven to raise your heart rates and adrenaline levels,[c] similar to what happens when you become aroused.
- Turn his body into an erotic canvas by using colorful finger paints. They are edible, so removing your masterpiece can be as enjoyable as creating it. You can purchase a body paint set in different flavors: mint, strawberry, lemon lime, and blueberry.

he want to kiss your breasts? Does he like how you touch him in that certain spot? And if he *were* here with you, where would he touch *you*?

- Don't forget your own pleasure. You may be the one doing the talking, but you can also touch yourself. If you feel confident, ask him to "guide" you. Go further and ask him if he is masturbating to the sound of your sexy voice.

Up to this point, you have explored the erotic elements and techniques of the inner circle of sexuality, where accepted rules and a prescribed course of action make it clear where the boundaries lie. Yet, another sphere exists. On your journey to the art of seduction, you are about to take a detour into a different arena, a world of pleasure where you can surrender to your wildest urges and indulge in the erotic realms of human nature in a very personal way. This world exists in Japan, where the participants know they are stepping outside their circle of obligations, and it is an accepted fact of life. According to anthropologist Ruth Benedict, "There is no reason not to indulge oneself but the two spheres belong apart."[8]

Indulge, if you dare. . . .

BATHHOUSE GAMES

In the days of Old Edo, when the government outlawed heated baths in all private houses in an effort to reduce the risk of fire, the *sento* or public bath was born.[9] There the male patron not only indulged in a pampered bath and massage, but also various kinds of sexual services with the young female attendants, *yuna*. *Sento* were popular for centuries and at one time nearly replaced the red-light districts.[10] Everyone knew of their existence and understood their proper place in society.

Today, secreted in the same quiet streets once immortalized in *ukiyoe* prints as the Yoshiwara of kimono-clad courtesans, you will find "soaplands." Many have the tone of theme parks with neon lights, stained glass windows, turrets, and battlements. One has a miniature putting green in the lobby for those who want a little sport before a soak and a rubdown. The girls often wear costumes—efficient nurses, coy schoolgirls, and trim airline attendants. Although sanctioned sex-selling was outlawed in 1956, there *are* loopholes. Soaplands avoid prosecution by promoting themselves as "assisted" bathhouses. Brothel guides as thick as telephone books are sold in convenience stores—along with the soap. In Japan it is not *what* you do, it is *how* and *where* you do it, especially regarding the pursuit of sexual pleasures.[11]

Considered an expensive indulgence, the soapland is always open, ready for the next customer whenever the urge to "get clean" strikes him. He can request a *shimei*, "nominated girl" or favorite.[12] She takes him to her room, takes off her clothes, then his. He sits on a stool while she soaps him until he is entirely covered with foam. She massages his body all over, then rinses off the soap. Smiling, she serves him chilled sake and washes his penis with a hot washcloth. Next, she invites him into the bath with her. Afterward she performs *awa-odori*, "lather dance." He lies on a waterbed or rubber mattress while she, swathed in

Sexy Sumo

Why not try a sexy version of the ancient art of sumo wrestling with your man? Sumo is combat between two people who can use nothing but their bodies. The famously hulking wrestlers, *sumotori*, are fast and agile. Many women find them incredibly sexy. Why? Because sumo embodies the fighting spirit. In sumo and in bed, it is the fight in the man as well as his penis that counts.

The wrestler begins by rubbing his hands together and brushing himself with a paper towel to symbolize cleansing mind and body before battle. He then tosses salt into the ring to purify and guard against injury. He claps once to alert the gods that a fight is about to begin. The opponents open their palms to show they have no hidden weapons, then strut and stare. They squat on the balls of their feet and face off in the fighting ring. Next, they lean forward and touch the knuckles of both hands to the ground. At the signal, they lunge forward, jockeying for a hold as they try to grapple their opponent out of the ring. The wrestlers wear only the *mawashi*, belt, a piece of fabric usually more than thirty feet long, tightly wrapped five or six times, and then cinched in back. It's rare for a *mawashi* to fall off, but if it does the wrestler automatically loses.

Though a single bout can be over in a flash (remind you of any past dates who couldn't wait?), the buildup can take ages (imagine the foreplay). In olden times, there was no limit on how long this buildup could continue—intriguing, isn't it? Touching, a little body friction between the two of you, no secret weapons, and wearing as little as possible. Sounds good, doesn't it? If he questions your motives and you don't get your way, you can simulate the heavy pounding of feet used in sumo called *shiko* to show your displeasure. And, if your clothing comes off, you automatically win, not lose.

milky suds and foamy bubbles, massages every part of him with every part of her. Finally, she rinses him off, "plays his flute," then ends the session with intercourse (men are required to wear condoms). Outside the dull, orange concrete building, the city of Tokyo bustles, oblivious to the heavy breathing of the man sweating in the steam.

The element of play found in these soaplands and "Turkish" bathhouses can add to your playtime pleasures. You can bring something new to your relationship that

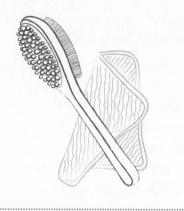

Use a brush and washcloth to give your man a hearty scrub in the bath

involves your erotic senses of smell, touch, even hearing. Put on your favorite costume for your man and give him a rubdown he won't forget. Undress, then get into the tub and let *him* soap you. When you're squeaky clean, perform a "bubble dance": cover yourself in soap then slide up and down on his nude body on a waterbed or a rubber mat. The scent of the soap turns you both on as you glide your foamy hands all over his body, while the refreshing sound of the water fills your ears, not to mention your husky voices moaning together in pleasure.

Hop in, the water is just right.

Bathing with Your Lover Tips

- Before you make love, suggest you share a bath. Prepare your bathroom beforehand with your favorite fluffy towels and scented candles, and with aromatic body wash or soap. Add a "theme" to get him all hot and sweaty and ready.

- Scent the bathwater. Two drops of patchouli oil and three drops of sandalwood oil will awaken sensuality. Add three drops of lavender oil to induce relaxation.

- Step in. The hot water will open the blood vessels near the skin's surface, making you both more responsive to touch. The combination of scents and warm-water sensations will completely prime your bodies—and your minds—for a truly sexual experience.

- Try sensual textures for washing: plush washcloth, natural sponge, big bath brush, gritty exfoliant.

- Even better, use your body. Soap yourself to a lather, and slowly cover every inch of his body with your own. You'll discover each other's hidden "hot spots."

- Bath vs. shower: you can expand your "playing" field to include the shower for different games.

- When you're in the shower, don't get out after washing. He's feeling all hot and steamy, especially after watching the bubbling beads of water slither down your breasts, hips, legs, and everywhere in between. You can make love if your heights match. Or stand on your tippy toes or position yourself on top of a small plastic stool, sliding your body up close to his, holding him close to you.

- Making love in a pool or hot tub, lake, or ocean is highly sensuous because it gives you both the feel of flying. Use the buoyancy you get in the water to have him prop you up at fun and interesting angles.

- Water doesn't hinder friction, though if the water temperature is cold, it may take some brisk rubbing or oral sex on your part to help him get an erection.

DANCE

Feeling sexy? More graceful? Put what you have learned into action. Dance! Japan's famous theatrical art of Kabuki, begun in 1603 when a shrine maiden named Okuni traveled to

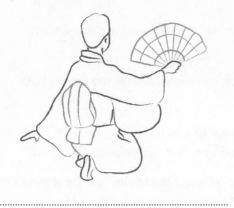

The dance of the geisha was a mesmerizing
mix of graceful hand motions and postures

Kyoto and, dressed in men's clothing while chanting Buddha's name, performed popular dances spiked with humor and eroticism. Men found her so exciting that women's Kabuki was banned. Years later, geisha developed famous dance skills of their own. When a geisha danced, her flowing limbs and graceful poses had the sensuality of liquid light. She looked elegantly alive, lifting up her head then lowering it, her feet delicately clad in white cotton *tabi*, her hands and her fan like the petals of an enchanted flower blowing in the breeze. A beautiful dancer is a mesmerizing one, no matter what her face or form.

Dance Tips

- The slow, controlled movements of the fixed patterns of a geisha's dance required a well-toned body as well as years of training. Keeping your body fit will make your dancing more graceful.

- When she dances, the geisha focuses on her relationship to the ground, being connected to the earth rather than the sky. Perform for your lover in either bare feet or high heels—both are *very* sexy.

- When geisha were still *maiko*, it was customary to flirt when dancing. If a guest became aroused and grabbed her, the girl would pretend to push him away while brushing up against him. Don't be afraid to use your body when you dance. Touch him and let him touch you. Your graceful movements, extended limbs and torso, the curve of your lovely derrière, all inflame desire.

- To make the moon round, a maiden of legend danced before the Palace of the Moon in a robe of pure white feathers. Feathers or fan(s) or silk scarves can make your dance more seductive. Use your imagination and see where they take you—and him.

- Geisha dances told stories, about the changing seasons, about going out to meet a lover, about older geisha reminiscing. They conveyed emotion through subtle head movements, hand gestures, and body language. Use different hand and body movements when you dance, keeping in mind that certain gestures will evoke different responses. Pay attention to see what turns your lover on.

APHRODISIAC ARTS

Dip into your secret arsenal in the art of seduction: aphrodisiacs. In the eighteenth century *ukiyoe* series "Glories of the Twelve Months" by Isoda Koryusai, a man is seen spying on his wife in the garden, eyeing her derrière as she does the laundry, then making love to her. In the same set of prints, a couple are enjoying themselves making love, the exquisitely exhausted wife asking her husband if he rubbed an aphrodisiac on his penis.[13] Aphrodisiacs are exotic, titillating, and even delicious.

During the era of the magnificent *tayu*, aphrodisiacs were part of her "secret cache" of drugs, medicines, and love potions to rev up the sexual energy of her customers for nightlong lovemaking. These included unsavory ingredients, such as extract of white dog liver, charred newts, and powdered dried lizard. If these weren't to the gentleman's taste, he could always choose herbal prescriptions,[14] including *jiogan,* "yellow earth pills," prepared from the roots of the *Rehmannia lutea,* a plant belonging to the figwort family;[15] lotus root; and *chomeigan,* an aphrodisiac thought to improve strength and endurance. *Kuroyaki,* a dark powder dissolved in sake, is still used today.[16] Certain nutritious foods, such as kelp and barley leaves, were understood to be beneficial for maintaining a powerful erection and sex drive. *Aojiru,* a greenish grass extract drink said to have an unpleasant taste, is a modern equivalent.

She also used substances to irritate the mucous membrane of the man's genitalia, intending to produce a warm, itching feeling similar to sexual arousal, and with it, an aphrodisiac effect. Unfortunately for the customer, his penis often became inflamed. In such a case, sandalwood oil soothed the resulting rashes. Because she herself epitomized sexual vigor, her female ejaculate was even drunk as an aphrodisiac and also thought to have rejuvenating properties to reverse the aging process.[17] Psychological aphrodisiacs included her outlandishly appealing clothing, including numerous "needles" or combs in her hair, her long, long kimono dragging behind her, and high, high *geta.*

For her *mabu,* secret lover, she more than likely employed a powder made from the slender, spiraled ivory tusk of the narwhal, a mysterious whale from the Arctic sea, often mistaken for that of the mythical

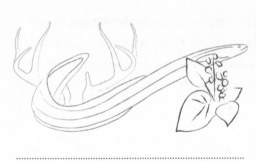

Deer antlers, horny goat weed, and eels were among the favored courtesan aphrodisiacs

Aphrodisiac Recipes

CHARBROILED OYSTERS CASANOVA*

⅓ cup butter or butter substitute • ⅔ Tbsp. finely chopped garlic • pinch or two of pepper • ⅛ cup or slightly less grated Parmesan cheese • ⅛ cup or slightly less grated Romano cheese • 11 Pacific oysters, on the half shell • ¼ cup finely chopped parsley

Heat the grill over medium high heat.

Melt the butter or butter substitute with the garlic and pepper in a large skillet.

Mix together the Parmesan and Romano cheeses in a small bowl.

Put the oysters on the grill. If you have trouble opening the oysters, put them on the grill a few minutes until they pop open. Remove the top shell, then drizzle the melted butter mixture on each oyster. Add a pinch of the combined cheeses to each oyster, then add a pinch of parsley.

Grill the oysters until they are hot, bubbly and puffed, about 8 minutes.

Casanova was reputed to eat dozens of oysters daily to increase his sexual prowess.

CHOCOLATE AMBROSIA LATTE

1 cup nonfat milk • ¼ (approximately 14 oz.) carton of silken tofu • 1 Tbsp. instant espresso powder • 2 Tbsp. cocoa • ¼ cup sugar • ½ teaspoon vanilla • ⅛ teaspoon almond extract • ½ cup crushed ice • chocolate whipped cream (for topping)

Mix milk, tofu, espresso powder, cocoa, sugar, vanilla, and almond extract in a blender until smooth. Add ice and blend again until it is a yummy frappé. Top with a luscious swirl of chocolate whipped cream. Serve cold. Makes 2 servings.

unicorn. Peniform mushrooms and hard deer antlers, powdered along with other herbs, were also believed to produce untold vigor and splendid, bone-hard erections. She also gave her lover horny goat weed to increase sperm production, stimulate the sensory nerves, and increase sexual desire. Eels were also a popular aphrodisiac. According to legend, when after

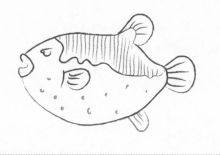

The tingling poison of the fugu blowfish
was considered a dangerous pleasure

numerous meetings and expensive gifts, a certain nobleman secured an evening with the most expensive *tayu*, he declared no one else in the pleasure quarters could indulge in eels on that day—*and* night.

The courtesan maintained her own sexual function by massaging herself with ginger oil. The warming, stimulating oil was known for its aphrodisiac qualities and fresh herbal smell, much less pungent than the root. Pleasing to both her and her lover was another drug she smeared onto a piece of paper, which she then wrapped around his penis. After inserting his penis into her vagina, the man waited a few moments for the aphrodisiac to melt. As it did so, his penis swelled, and at that moment the courtesan would flush slightly and slowly begin to move her limbs, then her hips, then her entire torso, until both reached the peak of satisfaction.[18]

Then there was, and still is, *fugu*. In Old Edo tales, beautiful heroines and lovers forbidden to marry would commit ritual suicide. Called *shinju,* lovers' suicide is an exquisitely tragic example of the Japanese fascination with beauty, pleasure, and death. So is *fugu*.

Fugu is a fish eaten as far back as the time of Japan's first official history in A.D. 720. The texture of the pearly white flesh is somewhere between crunchy and chewy. Bite a cool, firm slice and the palate tingles, a slight numbness spreads on the lips and tongue. But the ovaries, skin, liver, and intestines are lethal. They contain tetrodotoxin, a poison so potent the U.S. Food and Drug Administration warns that it can "produce rapid and violent death."[19] *Fugu* lovers are willing to take that chance to experience the sense of euphoria eating the fish induces in them. The key to successful preparation is the complete removal of the poisonous organs *before* the fins are cut off, grilled, and served in hot sake; the skin is removed from the flesh, which is poached and served; and paper-thin slices of *fugu* sashimi are arranged on the plate like the petals of a chrysanthemum, Japan's traditional funeral flower. A final course of *tetchiri*—*fugu* cooked in broth with vegetables, tofu, and noodles— brings the arousal from defying death to its peak. Then comes the aphrodisiac *pièce de résistance*: the *fugu* testes in a glass of hot sake. (Needless to say, do not attempt to prepare *fugu* on your own! *Fugu* chefs must be trained and licensed.)

You may not have access to the aphrodisiacs of the *tayu*, or even *want* them, but there are sensual and delicious foods that have an aphrodisiac-like effect for you both: oysters and chocolate.

OYSTERS

On Hekurajima, a small island near the Noto Peninsula, slim and tanned Japanese women, dressed only in loincloths with a rope around their waists, their bare breasts glistening, dive into the water for conches, garlands of edible seaweed, and oysters, often with pearls found nestled inside the shell. These mermaids have long known about the aphrodisiac quality of oysters. Oysters contain all the nutrients important to male fertility. They also have a smooth, moist texture, a briny taste, and a delicate aroma that can be very erotic. Their obvious resemblance to female genitalia spawned in Japan the usage of the word *bobokai*, "shell," as a metaphor for the vulva, and explains their link with love and romance in the West as well.

The Pacific oyster, originally from Japan, is the most widely cultured oyster in the world and is sold under a variety of names, including Kumamoto. It is creamier in flavor than the Atlantic variety, in which you can taste the saltiness of the ocean. Whatever their flavor, oysters are deep cupped, plump, and sweet, like your breasts. Good for him to nibble on. So, how do you eat an oyster? Here are some tips to make this erotic delicacy go down easily.

How to Eat Oysters Tips

- Like the taste of a woman, the subtle nuances in the flavor of oysters can only be discerned *au naturel*. Serve them grilled, raw with crushed ice and seaweed, or with a squirt of lemon or a sauce that does not mask the underlying taste.

- Hot sauce, horseradish, Worcestershire sauce, and seafood cocktail sauce are also good accompaniments to oysters.

If oysters don't send his sex-o-meter up, try chocolate. It is tasty, melty, and can be eaten in any shape that interests you. *Any* shape. Mmm . . .

CHOCOLATE

On Valentine's Day in Japan, women give chocolate to men, including their coworkers, bosses, male friends, brothers, father, husband, *and* their boyfriends. (Men give the women gifts on March 14, called White Day.) If a woman doesn't feel amorous toward a

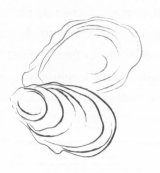

The look and texture of oysters make them primary among the list of sensual, sexual foods

man, e.g., her boss, she gives him *girichoco*, "obligation chocolate." To the man who makes her heart beat faster but who is not yet a prospective husband, she gives special gifts, such as neckties and clothes with chocolate. The chocolate she gives to her special man is called *honmeichoco*, "prospective winner chocolate." *Honmeichoco* is more expensive than *girichoco* and can be homemade.

Can chocolate make him fall in love with you? Chocolate is the perfect aphrodisiac because it contains substances called phenylethylamine and seratonin, mood-lifting agents that occur naturally in the brain. These cause a rapid mood change and a rise in blood pressure, increasing the heart rate and inducing feelings of well being, bordering on the euphoria he experiences with feelings of love, passion, and—dare you hope?—lust.

CHOCOLATE TIPS

• Eating chocolate with its luscious aroma, texture, sweetness, and flavor can also give him an immediate and substantial energy boost, increasing his stamina where it counts the most—in bed with you.

• The chocolate with the highest concentration of mood-enhancing substances is top-quality semisweet or bittersweet.

A FINAL WORD ON APHRODISIACS . . .

You don't have to stuff him with oysters, fill him up with chocolate, or make his mouth numb with *fugu*. The most powerful aphrodisiac is simple: attention, and plenty of it. Focus on your lover as if he were the only man in the room and in your life. Get him to talk. Engage in provocative questions, not bland conversation. If he says something funny or smart, or you like his cologne or his shirt, say so. This reassures him that you won't reject him. Geisha gave compliments all the time, and men knew they would be accepted for themselves. Let him know you have all the time he needs and you are in no hurry. If you want to see him again or don't want him to leave, drop hints. A geisha could coyly hand her customer another incense stick if she wanted him to stay, since her time was measured by its burning.

Sexy play is similar to the Japanese notion of *yoin*. *Yoin* is the sound a bell makes after it is struck. It is a "reverberation" in the sense of an overtone, a resonance. It implies that something you felt stimulated your imagination and caused a positive memory to linger.[20] A fleeting smile, a blush on your cheeks, a gentle touch, all produce *yoin*—and a sexier you. If you can instill *yoin* in his mind, he will remember you long after you leave the room.

By sharing a bath, good conversation, flirting, and games, you have broken through one of the most difficult parts of any couple bonding: communication. Conversation, touching, being spontaneous and playful, and letting yourself go all contribute to acquiring intimacy. Once you have formed this bond with him, you're ready for the next part of your journey: making love.

Chapter 7

SEEDING THE FLOWER AND TWIRLING THE STEM

"What in the devil are you doing?" the girl asked when she awakened and discovered a boy's penis inside her vagina thrusting as deeply as possible. "Do you know what you're doing to me?"

The young man replied in confusion, "Forgive me. I'll take it out immediately."

Pretending not to hear him, she said, "Heaven should punish you even more severely if you take it out."

Fukujuso, Sixteen Erotic Tales, 1778, Anonymous[1]

Tempting, teasing, and tantalizing, yet ever so tactful and polite, the sensual courtesan or geisha could bring any man to a peak of aroused anticipation. And, for the lucky guest to her liking, she knew where she would lead him next. *She* had the initiative; the choice was hers. Then, she let the prospect of mutual pleasure seduce them both.

You've mastered all the points of *kokono-tokoro*; you have *hari*; you are *iki*. You have hopelessly entangled that special someone in your web, developed a fun and interesting relationship so sensual he couldn't escape even if he wished, which, of course, he doesn't. If you are intrigued by the idea of becoming intimate with the man you've captured, the next step is for both of you to experience the ultimate: a richly satisfying sexual encounter. In this chapter, you will not only learn how to achieve orgasm and soar to new heights at his touch, but also explore the satisfying togetherness you feel afterward that makes your relationship complete. This is a hot chapter devoted exclusively to pleasure, his *and* yours. It is your essential guide to getting the most out of making love.

A COURTESAN'S VIEW OF SEX

Traditional Japan considered the pleasures of the body as a natural part of life. With her unique combination of refinement and earthiness, the courtesan was the "high priestess" of the celebration.

To assure success in love, the courtesan could follow the example of the past. Superstitious Heian court ladies believed there were lucky or unlucky days on which to have intercourse. To ensure that friendly gods would look favorably on the first night with a lover, the futon had to point due north-south with ashes of certain plants strewn around it, the room warmed by only certain types of wood in the brazier. Happy results also depended on the placement of doors, windows, and house altars, as well as the proper balance of *yin* (female, water, moon, north, and winter) and *yang* (male, fire, sun, south, and summer), which governed their daily lives. Exacting rules for style and color of dress enhanced a lady's allure. She even could turn to a sex manual written in 984 by Tanba no Yasuyori. Heian ladies believed the ideal man should be four to ten years older, but the courtesan had differ-ent priorities.

THE COURTESAN AND THE PENIS

The courtesan also benefited from Old Japan's delight in the penis. It took center stage in one version of the ancient Shinto creation myth, in which the world originated with a sex act. According to folklore, the god and goddess Izanagi and Izanami penetrated the ocean with a giant lance, producing the first island of Japan from the splash. Then, driving it into the belly of the world, they slid down to earth on this phallus-like symbol.[2] Male symbols for erotic enjoyment permeated every phase of Japanese life, from the phallus-shaped gilded hairpins of the prostitute, to the foot-long wooden phallus attached to the front of a sake cart that she could stroke or kiss for good luck, to the

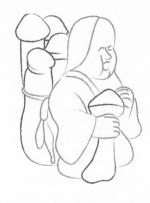

The mushroom-toting Okame is a folk goddess of sensuality and a good luck charm

erect mushrooms protruding upright from the backpack of the folk goddess of sensuality, Okame, a good luck charm even today.

Japanese fertility festivals also have fun with phallic symbols, where young women suck on penis-shaped candies and ride a penis-shaped seesaw.[3] Other remnants of the courtesan's world are the annual festival of the small town of Komaki, in which a six-foot-long wooden phallus is carried through the streets on men's shoulders, and the Tagata Jinja shrine, which showcases a large variety of phallus-shaped objects, both naturally occurring and man-made.

Nowhere was the phallus more celebrated than in the graphically descriptive, erotic *shunga*, where genitalia were the natural focus. Artists gave them detailed attention in portraying physical sensation and its culmination in a transportingly pleasurable orgasm—of both the happy participants and viewer. The earliest extant

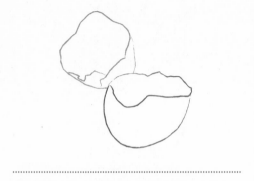

The contents of a raw egg were used for lubrication and as an aphrodisiac

example, a painted scroll called *The Phallic Contest*, depicts delighted women judging men endowed with enormous penises. In the ensuing orgy, the women invariably are more than a match for the men, who finally crawl away totally exhausted by their demands.[4] Such portrayals of the penis fantastically enlarged were an established convention. One master reputedly told his pupil that the penis was always depicted larger than life because if it were drawn in its natural size, it would hardly be worth looking at.[5]

That did not prevent the courtesan from making the most of the real thing. After first assessing whether her guest had a high and big nose, which she believed promised a big penis, she undressed him with several interesting terms of admiration rolling from her lips: *daijuisshi*, "eleventh finger"; *itaname*, "a floor polisher," for an extremely long penis; *uma*, "horse," for an extremely thick penis; and, *yohoko*, "a powerful lance."[6]

HER BODY HERSELF

The *maiko*'s initiation into the world of sex, and with it, her debut as a geisha, was a ceremonial one: *mizuage*. The word means "drawing from the water," from the notion that anything drawn from the water should be "fresh," as in a virgin.[7] A virgin was referred to as *arahachi*, a "new vase."[8] *Mizuage* was designed so the young *maiko* would not experience the uncouth manners of someone like the anonymous eighteenth-century libertine who boasted, "With a weapon like this, it would be hard not to break a new vase without causing pain. . . . "[9] The *okasan*, mama-san, would choose who would have the privilege of deflowering her. He would not be young, because a young man would be too rough. He had to be older, gentle, and sincere, although in the end, he also had to be the highest bidder.[10]

According to numerous writings on the subject, *mizuage* used to take seven days to perform. According to a modern-day account by a *shacho,* company president, the *mizuage* patron ". . . was something like a male honeybee . . . after his initial function was served, he had no further relation with the lady."[11] Each night during the defloration ritual, the man cracked open three eggs. He swallowed the yolks, which were considered aphrodisiacs, and rubbed the whites between the thighs of the *maiko*. Then, his hands lubricated by the slippery egg whites, he wiggled his fingers into her vagina, a little deeper each night. By the end of the week, the *maiko* was very relaxed and ready for her first sexual intercourse, the enjoyment of which was regarded as a parting gift to the guest.[12]

To openly mark this significant passage in her life, the new geisha wore a hairstyle called the "split peach," which included a piece of red silk visible in the split. This was most provocative, as it was public proof of defloration, making her change from *maiko* to geisha evident for all to see.[13]

For her part, the Yoshiwara courtesan used many different and evocative words when speaking about the delights of her body. She described her pubic hair as *shunso,* "spring grass"; her vulva as an *aodaisho,* "green snake," or an *akagai,* "ark shell"; her anus as the *uramon,* "rear door"; and her pudenda as a *gyokumon,* "royal gate."[14] She, and her patrons, also consulted the *Ukiyozoshi,* "Illustrated Manual of Eroticism," a 1686 compilation of knowledge concerning sexual pleasure. It had this to say about her genitals:

The royal gate is adequate for any dimensions, large or small; it is as adaptable as water which can accommodate itself to any contour. Further inside, there is a soft and flesh region resembling a tangerine slice and at the greatest depth one finds a small protrusion attached to the upper portion, like an extending finger. At this depth one encounters the region which is the source of love-juices capable of conveying the man's semen to the womb . . . women will gasp with ecstasy when a man's penis touches this region and their moans resemble the cooing of a nightingale enraptured with the delightful scent of plum blossoms mingling with a fine mist. An instrument of five to six inches is adequate for a proper royal gate.[15]

Although you may be wondering if your intended lover's genitals are as big as a horse's and yours look like a tangerine slice (put the mirror away and keep reading), your sex organs *are* unique. The better you understand his body and yours, the better, and more pleasurable, will be your lovemaking.

YOUR "ROYAL GATE" AND OTHER SENSUAL PARTS

The little mound over your pubic bone is your *mons veneris*, "mound of Venus." Your *vulva*, the external part of your genitalia, is the opening between the projecting parts of your sex organs. Around this are your "larger lips," *labia majora*, extending from your mound of Venus and tapering below your vaginal opening. Just inside them, and perhaps protruding a bit, are your "inner lips," *labia minora*, matching folds of delicate, hairless skin extending from directly above your clitoral head to your vaginal opening. They are pink and glisten with moisture.

Your *clitoris* or "female penis" is located below the top where your labia meet. It is made from the same kind of tissue as his penis and responds similarly when stroked. Unlike his penis, it doesn't have a hole, or *urethra*, running through it. (Your urinary opening is about one-half inch below your clitoris.) It is shaped like a pink root jutting out and is comparable to a little bean that swells when stimulated and becomes firm and responsive. It has a tiny glans and a little hood or foreskin called the *prepuce*.

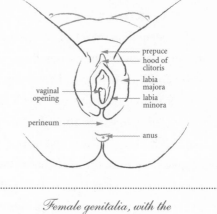

Female genitalia, with the erogenous zones labeled

Below the *urethral meatus* lies the entrance to your vagina—your largest female organ. It is three to four inches long, flexible, and made of folded muscle. The inside walls are covered with mucous membrane.

All of these parts are exquisitely sensual. Your labia are rich in nerve endings. You feel sexy sensations when they are sucked or gently tugged on. The texture, warmth, and wetness of your vagina are similar to that of your mouth. Deep kissing produces an immediate response that can take your breath away. The clitoris, your *wareme-chan*,[16] "dear little slit," exists for no other reason than to make you feel good. Its tiny hood, your pleasure "bean," *mame*, is not visible to his naked eye, so you can help him discover it by showing him how to massage this delicate spot in harmony with your heartbeat.

HIS "FLOOR POLISHER"

The *maiko* listened intently to her *onesan*, older geisha sister, when she advised her on the anatomy of the penis. "Only when he is hard and angry," she told her, "the skin taut like a bow string and the purple head straining like a fish out of water, can you begin."[17] What does this mean in modern terms? You'll see.

Penis size varies, though there is no correlation between its size and that of other body parts. Your lover's flaccid penis may be as short as two inches or as long as seven; erect, it may range from under four inches to over ten. It contains no muscle or bone. When he becomes aroused by your presence, blood flows into the erectile tissue, causing it to swell and stiffen so the penis can easily penetrate your vagina. Most men claim an extra inch or two for their penis. What he does with it, not the size, is what matters.

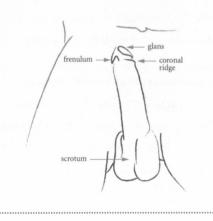

Male genitalia, with the erogenous zones labeled

His penis consists of a shaft and a head. The *coronal ridge* is the area where the head meets the shaft. If he is circumcised, this is where the operation was performed. Inside the shaft is his urethra, which carries semen or urine and which opens outside his body through a tiny slit in the mushroom-like top of the head, called the *glans*. When his penis is erect, it makes a bulging ridge that you can run your finger along. Beneath his penis is his *scrotum*, the external pouch of skin holding his *testicles*. His testicles, commonly called his "balls," are where his sperm is made and stored for ejaculation. They move constantly to prevent them from getting too hot. In most men, one testicle hangs lower than the other to keep them from crushing each other. A man with one testicle can function as efficiently as a man with two. The *perineum* is the erogenous zone located between the base of his testicles and his anus.

The courtesan made the most of her expert knowledge about the penis and its amazing sensitivity to the touch. With a little practice and attention, you can do what she did. The underside of your lover's erect penis is more sensitive then the upper side. The head and the ridge around its base are even more sensitive. The perineum is rich in nerve endings and very sensitive to sexual stimulation. He enjoys having you touch or stroke this area. Then, there is the skin of the *frenulum*. An inverted V-shaped spot located where the head and shaft meet, it faces away from his body. It is his most erotic area. Making him hot is in your hands, and when he's hot, you'll have your way.

Gentleness and sensitivity are important for both you and your lover. Direct stimulation on your "love bean" is not only uncomfortable, it can even be painful. Some women worry about vaginal size. If you think you're too small and intercourse may be painful, it's more likely not due to your size but to your inability to relax or a tough hymen (the fold of mucous membrane partly closing the orifice of the vagina). If his penis feels loose in your vagina, switch to a position where your thighs are pressed tightly together. If your vagina is tight, it will give him extra intense feelings. Be aware that his testicles are the most sensitive part of his anatomy because they have nothing to protect them. Pressure on a testis is highly painful to him. The perineum is also highly sensitive and needs careful handling. Making love is an emotionally vulnerable time. If you have difficulties with how you touch each other, share them when you are *not* naked in bed.

Condoms

When the *oiran* took her guest's penis in her hand, more than likely she put a sheath on his organ. With their combined sensuality, refinement, and practicality, it was the Japanese who first developed a covering for the penis to serve the dual purpose of preventing semen from entering the womb and intensifying enjoyment of the act of copulation. Most pleasurable to both courtesan and guest was a condom with "rings" added to the surface of the sheath, including raised corrugations and comb-like or prickly protuberances made from different materials, and later from specially hardened rubber. The idea was to bring the genitals closer together for mutual enjoyment, whatever the size of their sex organs. The Japanese have various words for condom: *sakku*, "sac," *gomu*, "gum," *kondomu*, "condom," even *Kondo-san*, "Mr. Condom."

Condom materials over the years have included snakeskin, silk, paper, leather, linen, tortoise shell, sheep bladders, and rubber. Today you can choose latex (the most durable available and, if used correctly, protective against pregnancy and STDs), polyurethane (which blocks sperm and most viruses and is thinner than latex so it transmits heat better, making sex feel more natural to both of you), or animal membrane (which prevents pregnancy but does not protect against most sexually transmitted diseases).

Always put the condom on his penis yourself. You can trust yourself. You know you will put it on right. In modern Japan, "skin ladies," *sukin redi*, sell condoms door-to-door to help couples practice contraception, *hinin*. Buy the right size. In Japan, ads for *gaijin*-sized, "foreigner-sized," condoms are a big hit. He will appreciate it when you don't assume that "one size fits all."

HIS BODY TIPS

- Kiss your man's penis often. He will love you for it.

- The typical Japanese penis points to the right. Which way does your man's penis point? Not sure? Check it out. Understanding how to handle his penis, making it pulsate or ejaculate, is a major part of being in harmony with your lover. Learn to play with his penis skillfully, both with your hands *and* with your mouth.

- Don't bend his erect penis or get him into a sexual position where his penis could get bent by accident. This can happen when you are on top and if you are careless near orgasm, or, if you put him in you when he is not fully stiff and you move too quickly. It is possible to fracture one of the two hydraulics contained in his shaft.

- Don't comment on his penis size except favorably. What your eyes or face say is important to him. React positively, as the courtesan learned to tell men only what they wanted to hear.

FOREPLAY

Don't worry. I'll be a butterfly in the next life, and I'll come back and tickle you on the sleeve.

Shioda Ryohei, *Higuchi Ichiyo Kenkyu*, p. 701[18]

In *The Tale of Genji*, Lady Higekuro emptied the ashes of a brazier onto her husband's head to prevent him from visiting a rival. Her jealous display shows the importance of the act of love to these sensual women. So do the ideograms of the word *seiko*, "sex": *sei*, "heart" and "life," and *ko*, "mixing together." That tells us that everything in life mingled with the affairs of the heart, and *that* means that Heian ladies, not to mention the geisha and courtesans of later times, made use of it all in the art of foreplay. Much time was spent creating a web of love-play through conversation and the display of musical and choreographic accomplishment. Only after having entrapped a man did the ladies of old Japan turn to more physical enticements. Erotic preliminaries did not last a mere hour or two, but might stretch into days, weeks, or months before crossing the threshold to full intimacy. Now that you know how to entice, you can enjoy foreplay in the same manner. And, you won't have to go to the lengths of Lady Higekuro.

The greatest artist of foreplay was the courtesan. When she peeked over her fan and locked eyes with her lover, sparks flew. Wearing only a silk slip, *nagajuban*, under her kimono to lightly cover her breasts, she would ignite the flame by bending toward him, allowing the fold of her kimono to open. Show your cleavage—or your back, your shoulder, a length of leg through a slit skirt. Try going braless. The feel of the fabric against your nipples will stimulate them to erectness, and the sight of your hard cherry buds will turn him on. Put erotic thoughts into his mind. The courtesan made *shunga* available to her guest awaiting her entrance, putting before his eyes the act of love as a progression, from the immediate pleasure of masturbation to other preludes—lovers stroking each other's breasts or caressing one another's genitals. Not touching can be provocative. Your man is stimulated visually. Imagining *all* of your body, from seeing *part* of it or being made to *think* of it, arouses him. Doing these things arouses *you*. Start with a smoldering glance. . . .

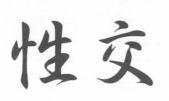

The Japanese word for "sex" is seiko, combining "heart/life" with "mixing together"

From visual enticement to physical arousal, the courtesan prided herself in the arts of massage, touch, and embrace, clothed and unclothed. She used her knowledge of the "sex points," beginning at his navel and continuing directly above and below it, moving to his chest, lips, forehead, back of his head, and the back of his neck in such a way as to provide the greatest pleasure for her partner. She could drive a man crazy with the touch of her fingers, and then, with her feet in dainty white tabi or perhaps with her bare toes, massage his crotch. Then, unclothed, she explored these erogenous zones. Slowly, precisely, with a technique somewhere between massage and making him squirm with pleasure, teasing and tantalizing him to orgasm from a simple touch of her fingers, she brought her lover to a state of enlightenment through sex.

Making love should begin with play and seduction, and continue until your minds and spirits are harmonious. Only then, holding each other, whispering words of passion, should you make love. You becoming moist with desire, his penis hard with longing for you—these are your goals. From foreplay to making love, you don't have to go about it in a repetitious, predictable manner. His whole body is an erogenous zone, so find every way you can to enjoy it. Teasing and touching, slow and quick, caressing and grasping, naughty and smoldering, there is no single path. Seduction is about anticipation.

What if he won't wait, you ask? He will. He's as interested as you are and wants more foreplay than he's getting. He likes it because it feels good and the extra anticipation makes him feel his orgasm more intensely. The longer and stronger his orgasm, the more your delight. Prolonging *his* excitement also causes *you* to build more excitement, so when you climax, you also experience a greater sense of release and pleasure.

FOREPLAY TIPS

- In many *shunga*, the lovers stimulate their lovemaking by keeping their eyes open. Sweep your eyes upward, then downward, looking at each other in a saucy manner when you kiss. This opens your minds to the emotional side of physical love.

- If you want to soothe him, give him a refreshing scalp massage, firmly rubbing each pressure point in circular motions. He will enter a relaxed, almost hypnotic state of mind and be willing to do just about anything you desire. *Anything*.

- Make him the sexy voyeur of his own seduction. Stand in front of a mirror and slowly undress him so he can see what *you* are doing to *him* as the clothing falls away. Expect him to rise to the occasion.

- Do as the playful lovers in the *shunga* do and leave on one piece of clothing. "Nearly naked" is arousing because it keeps the mystery alive. And *him* wanting to see what he can't have. Not yet. Involve all your body in your game. Hold him close with one hand and grab his cute butt with the other while you press against him.

- Let *his* imagination do some of the work for you. Touch your lover clothed. Keeping your clothes on heightens your own anticipation and adds a bit of mystery for him about what is underneath.

Had enough? You'll know when he is aroused. He can't help but be enchanted by the sight, smell, and taste of you. Now the real fun begins: your energetic, passionate, and exciting sexual adventure. That's where this whole journey is leading, isn't it?

MAKING LOVE

> You and I together, we're like an egg yolk: as for me I'm the white part, and I embrace you tightly![19]

Experiencing physical love, many a courtesan murmured this lyrical expression from Japanese folklore to her lover: *hitosame no nure ni*, "once they were bedewed with rain."[20] Erotic love in Old Edo was an art practiced with extreme care and according to careful guidelines, as discussed in *An Illustrated Manual of Eroticism* by Yoshida Hanbei, a 1686 compilation of knowledge concerning sexual pleasure. Courtesans' bedroom techniques were highly developed. They placed the greatest value on their sensations while making love, and gave every possible assistance toward arousing and sustaining the sexual feelings of their partners.

"PENIS PLAY"

Erotic "penis play" is about touch, from lightly kissing his genitals to arousing caresses. Or, if you are artistically inclined, you can follow the example of the *oiran* in the *shunga* book *Young Pine Saplings* by Katsushika Hokusai (1760–1849) who engages in erotic play by writing on her man's penis with a paintbrush.[21] However you enjoy it, think of "penis play" as awakening your lover to the urges of nature, the building of storm clouds to nurture a certain flower—you. Flirt with his penis. Tease it, play with it, then be wanton, naughty, and daring. Like a geisha flicking her fan, you can change your mood. Be sensitive, silly, tender, caring. Don't rush. Move slowly,

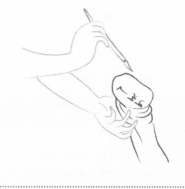

"Penis painting," as imagined in an erotic woodblock print

yet with seductive purpose. Think about the gentle fluttering of the butterfly, the graceful sway of the geisha's head, or the swish of her long kimono sleeves sweeping the tatami. Savor his penis, guiding him to a blissful state by varying your caresses.

PENIS PLAY TIPS

- Fondling is an art, like the hand movements of a *maiko* performing the dance called *Nanoha*, the story of the butterfly and the plum blossom.

- *Te o dasu*, "put out your hand," as in "make the first move." Be playful. Stick your hand in his pocket and touch his penis through his pants, pretending you're looking for change. When he is hard, whisper something naughty in his ear.

- Wrap your arms around him and run your hands down his back and buttocks. Move your fingers gently to the base of his spine. Rest your fingertips above the crack in his buttocks and press into the bone. Then, lightly stroke his perineum with your fingertips. Slide your hands to his crotch. Softly gather his genitals in one hand, and with great care, caress his groin with the other. His knees will buckle with pleasure, and he will be hard where you want it.

- Smooth some lubricant on his penis and stroke it in a swirling motion. You will ignite nerve endings he didn't know he has.

- Caress his ultrasensitive frenulum. You will feel it actually grow hot and even tingle a little or vibrate from the increased blood flow.

- Like the soft wind swaying the willows, blow kisses across his penis. Breathe on it lightly, whisper, tickle, then kiss it gently.

- Move your fingers to his erect penis. Hold it near the tip, then slide toward the base to make the skin taut to pleasurably expose and tighten the engorged head. Heighten the sensation with short, light, back and forth motions of your fingertips.

- The shaft of his penis is the softest part of his anatomy. The skin is fine and delicate like the mist hovering around Mount Fuji. Gently pump with your hand, bringing him just short of ejaculation. By building up his anticipation, you will give him great pleasure and arouse him tremendously.

- If he starts to climax and begins thrusting, don't drop your hand and leave him hanging. Relax him slowly with a gentle massage from the base of his penis to its head. If you want him to climax in you, slow him down by squeezing under the head of his penis. This will stifle his urge until you can get into your favorite position. Avoid touching the head and tip, which will have become supersensitive.

- Close your eyes or leave them open. Whichever way you find harmony with his penis, make certain you relay your admiration for his magnificent mushroom with loving words, breathy sighs, and moans.

- Talk is sexy. Treat your lover to *sumata*, a courtesan's technique for prolonging anticipation:[22] Both nude, he would lie on top with his penis between her legs as she engaged in witty sexual repartee while squeezing her legs together tightly, trapping him between her thighs. The warmth and naughty talk aroused him to rock his hips from side to side, making his *chinko*, penis, even harder. He was ready for action when she finished.

• Try *paizuri*:[23] Have him thrust his penis between your breasts as you squeeze them together tightly around him. Encourage him to go slowly and enjoy the sensation as you move your breasts up and down.

Ready to up the stakes? It is time for oral sex, up close, and oh so personal.

ORAL SEX

Slowly, as if it is a delicious thing to you, take the head in your mouth . . . look up and meet his gaze. Oh yes, he will be watching. . . .

Instructional guide from a geisha to a *maiko*[24]

The young *maiko* gazed upon the *shunga* depicting a naked woman about to put her lover's penis into her mouth. She shivered with delight, looking forward to the day she would practice this *gei* to please *her* lover. To see such a print was a rare treat. Although many showed a man enjoying a woman's vulva, his eyes open with pleasure and a smile on his lips, few showed a woman giving oral sex to a man. Yet, *shakuhachi o fuku*, "blowing the flute," was a prized skill of the geisha and the *oiran*. Even today, hostess clubs offer private rooms where a woman will perform on the *shakuhachi*, and where oral sex is also called *kyande*, "candy." Patrons can enjoy what is popularly called *hamonika*, oral sex on the woman, but

Semen

In *shunga*, lovers are usually depicted with legs entwined and kimonos tangled around them. Scraps of crumpled paper allude to the man's ejaculation of semen, and also to the lovers' extravagance. Paper was very expensive and precious. His semen also was precious, as the heroine in Ihara Saikaku's seventeenth-century novel *The Life of a Woman Captivated by Sensuality* (also known as *Life of an Amorous Woman*) noted: "My only wish would be to see the amorous stream [semen] emulate this flowing current by never running dry."[b] He may enjoy watching his semen shoot out of his penis or prefer you to swallow it. "Oh, yes, swallow the ocean spume or the balance (of nature) is disturbed,"[c] urged the geisha to her little geisha sister. Both can be very sexy, but the choice should be yours.

SEMEN TIPS

- If you choose to let him eject semen into your mouth, you can swallow it or keep a cloth or napkin nearby to dispose of it discreetly. If he ejaculates more than twice during lovemaking for a couple of days, his semen may taste sour or acidic.
- If you spill semen over each other, gently massage it into your skin. The pollen odor is itself an aphrodisiac. Rub it on your face and breasts. It is whispered that rubbing her lover's semen made a geisha's skin shine.
- You can get spilled semen out of your clothing, furnishings, or sheets either with a stiff brush after the stain has dried, or with a diluted solution of sodium bicarbonate.
- He ejaculates only about a teaspoon of semen if he is between the ages of eighteen and thirty-six. Older men eject less. Semen contains ten calories in a tablespoon and thirty-two different chemicals.
- A word of caution: Swallowing semen during oral sex if he is HIV-infected has been known to transmit the deadly virus.

not engage in *honban*, a slang word for intercourse used when bragging about one's sexual exploits.[25]

Enjoying his penis alone is called fellatio. "Oral sex" partakes of his penis, scrotum, and/or perineum. You can begin when his penis is flaccid and stimulate him to erection. It is an important tool in your art of seduction, a skill in itself which will help you engage in more fulfilling lovemaking. Intercourse aside, genital kissing and touching are the most passionate and intimate acts of erotic communication that you can have. Make your experiences special by varying your speed and rhythm to the soft, romantic sound of the *shakuhachi*, wooden flute, or other music special to you both. Find out what he likes best— not by asking him, but by showing him—and harmonize your oral desires with his. What is most important is that you *enjoy* giving him oral sex. Whatever you do down there, as long as you don't hurt him, he'll love you for it. And, like the geisha after her debut, when she is called *shinbana*, "new flower," *you* will be filled with anticipation and energy for what comes after. Be playful and have fun!

BEFORE ORAL SEX TIPS

- "Playing his flute" requires complete cleanliness, and washing is a wonderfully seductive opportunity to build anticipation. With soap and warm water, tenderly wash his penis. Go slowly, and take care not to overstimulate his supersensitive areas so that he becomes aroused at your touch, but does not lose control.

- Do things that you both find arousing. Let your lover enjoy the sight of you touching him. Let him see, feel, even hear your seduction—you may wish to talk to his penis as you attend to it.

- When you have finished, dry him with a soft towel and move to kissing his perineum and scrotum. Hold the base of his penis with one hand so that it stands vertically and you control the situation.

GIVING HIM ORAL SEX

> Impossible! I took his *matsuke* [penis] in my mouth until my jaw ached. I
> sucked him until my eyes watered.[26]

As you take your lover gently into your mouth, think of oral sex as an artfully arranged
kaiseki, an elegant meal, each part of him a delicious dish. Position yourself comfortably so
you're sitting or kneeling to the side, almost perpendicular to his pelvis. An ice cube or a
mint in your mouth will give extra stimulation. Cup your hand around his penis, creating
a sexy cover. Then kiss the part that is exposed. Your hand will trap your breath and make
him feel delightfully hot.

Next, kiss the head lightly. Lick it and the tiny urethra opening with the tip of
your tongue. Then hold it in your mouth, surrounding the ridge with your lips. With your
lips a perfect "O," move up and down or let
him move in and out, while your fingers play
lightly on his perineum and scrotum. This
is the basic genital to mouth maneuver he is
expecting—and enjoys. The wise courtesan
could sense if she was causing discomfort
with her teeth or by stroking too quickly or
too slowly. You can tell if your man is enjoying great pleasure if he caresses your hair
or your face, or moves your head in rhythm
with his own movements.

Oral sex will not only arouse him

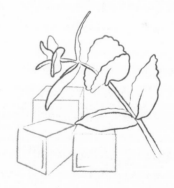

*Use mint or an ice cube to provide
extra stimulation during oral sex*

More Playful Sex Techniques

- The Japanese word for tongue is *shita*. Give him a tongue bath. Go over every inch of him, tied up if he likes it. Start with his back and cute butt, then turn him over and cover his chest, down to his penis until he is ready for action. You can heat him up even more by doing it again—with slow, graceful strokes of your open vulva.

- The summer heat is stifling along Kyoto's River Kamo. A geisha cools her lover by blowing on his skin. It's a nice follow up to a tongue bath—yours or his. For broader coverage, use water or lotion. Air from your lips, or even a hair dryer with the heat turned off, on wet, sensitive insides of the elbows, wrists, knees, and genital areas will create a contrast of warm and cold that can turn you both on.

- Some of the most underrated erogenous zones on your body lie in areas you might consider too ticklish to touch. Geisha nibble their food, which is always served bite-sized. You can gently nibble his penis, fingers, and ears; however, don't have an orgasm with body parts in your mouth. You can bite hard without realizing it. Stimulate his body inside and out. Slide your hand up to his chest and make circular movements around his nipples or use a finger in his anus to massage his prostate.

- A favorite sucking technique of the courtesan was a swirling motion going up and down, and sideways. As you move up and down his shaft—your lips open like budding flowers—turn your head a bit from side to side so your tongue follows a corkscrew pattern. Lick at his frenulum for a few seconds before moving all the way up to the top of his penis.

- Hum. With the tip of his erect penis into your mouth, make a low noise in the back of your throat. The vibrations give extra stimulation. Meanwhile, caress the bottom of his shaft and his testicles.

but also promote genital lubrication. Wetness is vital to intercourse. If he secretes while you are fondling him, trace your fingertip in a rotary motion to spread it around the head, enhancing his pleasurable sensations while preparing his penis for making love to you. You can also use your own or his saliva. The courtesan of Kyoto's Shimabara quarter often had help from the customer himself when " . . . he tried to insert his penis into her but because his penis was exceptionally large he did not succeed . . . he moistened it with his own saliva several times. . . ."[27]

SUCKING AND TONGUE TIPS

- An old Yoshiwara saying is ". . . everything can be done with lip service, even love."[28] In the flowers-and-willows world, the geisha was touted as an *artiste*, while the courtesan was considered a "flower" who offered garden variety sexual favors,[29] although both were known to grant a customer oral pleasures.

- Put yourself in the mood. Think of it as a pleasure that leads to more pleasure. Sucking is the most important thing you can learn to please him. Build your speed, harmonizing with his rhythm as well as his desire. You want to feel his emotions.

- Run your tongue around the head as if you're savoring the sweetness of red bean cakes, then flick it back and forth and all around his supersensitive frenulum. Don't worry about your tongue getting tired. It is the strongest muscle in your body.

- Stroke him while you're sucking. Run your hands over his inner thighs and listen to him moan.

- Then, like the bamboo rustling outside the geisha teahouse, run your tongue along his perineum for extra sensations that will make him love you forever.

- Taste his juices as if they were refreshing, delicious raindrops wetting your lips.

- Getting pubic hair in your mouth is normal. The courtesan would send her long, long sleeve billowing up in a graceful gesture to distract him as she took the hairs out of her mouth before continuing. Follow her example. He will be too turned on to notice.

- His penis, like a delicious *shiitake* mushroom, is a delicacy to be treated with respect. Your manicure may be pretty to look at, but sharp nails can ruin the night. Keep your teeth away, or very lightly rub them against him while sucking.

DEEP THROAT TIPS

- The *onesan*, older geisha sister, told her little geisha sister to " . . . search out the sweet tears of honey with your tongue as you slide him deep in your mouth."[30] To deep throat him (allowing the tip of his penis to touch your throat), take his penis down slowly, gradually until you can accommodate him easily. Try swallowing when it reaches the back of your throat. It tickles.

- Take a deep breath beforehand to relax your throat muscles. Or, direct his penis to one side of your mouth or cheek to avoid direct contact into your throat. In this way, you avoid triggering your gag reflex.

- His large penis will stretch your mouth. Use lip balm to prevent your lips from cracking and cover your teeth with your lips to protect his sensitive skin.

- Female-oriented *manga,* comics, always present men's genitals humorously as bananas, sausages, cucumbers or vibrators, but streaming with sexual fluids. He may ejaculate into your mouth, but his semen is clean and harmless. If you don't want him to ejaculate, stop just short of orgasm, then shift his penis to your breasts or your face.

- Not all men climax during oral sex. If he does, try after-orgasm genital kissing or sucking or massaging his penis gently for a few minutes. Go very carefully on the sensitive head. Concentrate on the base or midsection instead. If your man is so virile he can't take the lightest genital kissing or caressing before ejaculating, save this oral sex technique until he needs a new erection.

Genital kisses can greatly enhance sexual intimacy if you are in harmony about each other's expectations. That's why playing the flute well was one of the most treasured gifts in the art of the courtesan. With the techniques you have learned, you can give your man one of the most loving gestures in the entire sexual experience. The best way to experience oral sex, whether or not you reach orgasm, is to take turns. Don't be shy about asking him to do the same for you.

That's right. Now it is *your* turn.

ORAL SEX FOR YOU

Numerous *shunga* celebrate men engaged in *omonkuu*, "cunnilingus,"[31] partaking of the female essence from the source, lapping up the invigorating tonic as the excess juices dripped down a woman's parted thighs to collect in a sake cup. The slip of red silk in the newly initiated courtesan's split-peach hairstyle simulated her pink genital flesh, visually enticing a man to taste her "royal gate." While considered particularly beneficial to men, it is clear that the courtesans of Old Edo also enjoyed this sensual pleasure.

How you entice your man to drink from your fountain can be just as creative, from wearing split panties to scented underwear. Keep in mind that the hot, salty smell of your natural bouquet when you are sexually aroused turns him on, but sweat, body odor build-up, and the smell of feminine hygiene products will turn him off. You must be completely clean. Don't be afraid to tell him what pleases you the most. If you're shy about having him kiss you *asoko*, "down there," try oral sex in the dark.

WHEN HE GIVES YOU ORAL SEX TIPS

- The courtesan enhanced her sexual experience by watching what her lover was doing to her. Lie on your back with a pillow supporting your head as your lover rests your buttocks and lower back upon his upper thighs. When he bends over, your buttocks should be within reach of his mouth, while you get a good view.

- Lie on the edge of a low table like those found in every geisha teahouse and spread your legs wide. He kneels before you, giving him full control, and you complete pleasure. He begins by kissing your mons veneris, opens the outer lips of your vulva with his fingers, then caresses your blood-engorged inner lips with his tongue. Pleasurable sensations run through you as he sweeps his tongue up and down, touching the glands on either side of the vaginal entrance (they secrete a lubricating mucus during arousal), thrusting into your vagina, pulling out, then repeating his moves, his own natural rhythm in harmony with yours.

- A famous *shunga* depicts a close-up of a man licking a woman's clitoris. The word for "leech" engraved in the corner alludes to his ardor. You won't be able to lie still as he licks upward from the base of your clitoral shaft, alternating caresses between your clitoris and vulva and tickling you like a butterfly.

- When you are aroused, the wall of your vagina produces a generous liquid. If a courtesan wanted to save her ejaculation for herself, she used a specially made *heikonoinho*, dildo,[32] to capture it. If you're worried about secretions during oral sex (his or yours), specially designed latex barriers are available for use while performing cunnilingus and rimming (oral/anal sex).

LUBRICANTS

A passage in *Eiga Asobi Nidai Otoko,* the story of a libertine published in 1755, explained the importance of lubricant to the courtesan:

> . . . now I understand why he asked for lubricating paper. Thus, he picked up the paper and the *nerigi* [a powder-white lubricant produced from dried sea algae and mallow roots], which lay beside the bed, moistening them until they were soft enough for carefully coating his instrument. Then he guided it toward the "gate," intending to insert it slowly and gently. To his great surprise his "weapon" slid toward its destination without the slightest resistance like a person's foot slipping into moist mud.[33]

Lubricant is the most important tool in your art of lovemaking. When you are about to have intercourse, dry friction will get you nowhere. But a lubricant can boost your sexual experience. It acts like a bridge that transfers—and increases—the pleasurable sensations you feel on your skin deep down to your nerve endings. When you are comfortably wet, he will be able to glide then thrust more vigorously without hurting you, making both of you less inhibited, feel more intensely, and enhancing your climax.

Geisha decorated the teahouse with flowers to harmonize with the time of year:

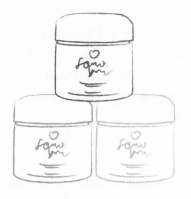

Lubricants come in jars, bottles, or tubes and can significantly boost sensation during sex

plum, peach, and cherry blossoms in the spring, and wisteria and lotus blossoms in the summer. Keep your lubricant in a pretty pump bottle and place it on your nightstand next to seasonal flowers to add a touch of elegance to an important part of your lovemaking.

Lubricant Tips

- The excited vagina is set for friction. If you are not there yet, enjoy more foreplay. If you are *too* wet (which may happen on the Pill) dry gently with a handkerchief-wrapped finger (not tissues—they are made of wood fibers and shred easily).

- The best sexual lubricant is saliva—yours or your lover's.

- Silicone lotion mimics your natural wetness and doesn't evaporate as quickly as other artificial lubes. You can use it underwater in hot tubs, bathtubs, and pools.

- Use only water-based lubes. They are tasteless and odorless, wash out of your body easily, and are less likely to provoke infection or allergic reaction. If one dries out while you are using it, you can reactivate it with a little water or saliva. Some have a gel-like texture, which is great for anal intercourse, and come in a convenient pump dispenser.

Fit for the Ride 1

How do you prepare for good sex? Here are some "sexercises" to get you ready.

- Before sex, loosen up and get rid of tension with the Japanese woman's *shiatsu* method for stimulating reflexes linked to the uterus: Cross your left foot over your right knee; with your right hand, press the indentations between your anklebone and heel for ten seconds. Switch feet. Repeat.

- Practice the "pubic squeeze": Suck in your stomach as far as it will go, then tighten your lower abdominal muscles. Hold for a few seconds, relax, repeat. This can be done lying on your bed, sitting at your desk, even watching television. He will never know when you're doing it, but you *both* will know the difference at the moment of climax.

- Geisha slept on their backs on the *tatami*. Lie on your back on the floor, legs together and knees straight, arms alongside your body with your palms downward. Perform your pelvic thrust or pubic squeeze as discussed. You can vary it by performing the same exercises with your legs spread apart.

- The very important "gluteal squeeze" enables you to attain a full vaginal orgasm by tensing and relaxing your buttocks to directly move your vagina forward and backward. It's not easy, so keep practicing! Stand tall with heels touching; tighten and squeeze your buttocks together while forcing your pubic area forward. At the same time, squeeze your thighs together and contract the muscles of your vagina. Hold for a count of eight, then relax, for five repetitions. The results are worth the effort.

- Geisha spent a lot of time sitting on their heels. Sit back on your heels, bend forward at the waist as far as possible, sliding the backs of your hands on the floor beside your feet as you place your face on the floor. Raise your torso to the starting position, then repeat, doing two sets of five repetitions.

- For a natural product, try honey—it washes off easily and is harmless.

- Lubes to avoid: Petroleum jelly is greasy, reduces sensation, leaves an unpleasant feel, and traps infection-causing bacteria. Moisturizers, like massage oil and mineral oil, stain sheets and break down the latex in condoms, which exposes you

Fit for the Ride 2

Let's not forget the man in your life. In Japan, men have always engaged in the study of martial arts and Bushido, the "Way of the Warrior," which, in the end, is all about mental endurance and control. Here are some exercises specifically for your man that will help increase his control during sex.

- The gluteal squeeze for him: He makes a conscious effort to extend and raise the penis when tensing the buttocks and forcing his genital region forward. The resulting muscular action will put more "feel" into the sex act and heighten his pleasure as well as yours.
- Penis contraction. He sits on the floor with knees bent and feet flat on the floor. Placing his hands on the floor behind his buttocks, he concentrates on his penis, trying as hard as possible to contract the muscles that raise it. Hold for a count of eight, then relax.

to STDs or pregnancy. Some lubes have nonoxynol-9, which can irritate your vagina and make sex uncomfortable. Flavored or colored lubes usually contain irritating chemicals.

"HOW SHALL I LOVE THEE?"

In addition to anal sex, fellatio, and cunnilingus, the courtesan counted in her repertoire *shijuhachi te*, forty-eight positions for intercourse, following the traditional number of falls of the sumo wrestler. She received instructions on lovemaking from guides of the time, including *Takisuka*, "Lighting the Flame," and *Moekui*, "Stoking the Fire." Published in 1677 by an unknown author, both guides borrowed from *The Mystic Master of the Grotto* by Dong Xuan Zi, the director of the Imperial School of Chinese Medicine during the Tang Dynasty (618–907). Writing with colorful language, he advocated pushing the "jade stalk" down and letting it move to and fro over the "lute strings" like a saw, as if prying open an oyster to obtain the precious pearl shining inside.

The courtesan took great pride in her skill. A paramour once wrote:

. . . her amorous behavior is so diversified that it is impossible to list details. One thing which she prefers is to grasp the man's penis and to kiss his lips frequently. When the penis enters her royal gate, she clasps the man tightly and as he thrusts more quickly she sighs deeply, with her body becoming tense and with her head moving from left to right so that she never remains absolutely still.[34]

Warm and moist, aching for him, this is the moment you have dreamed of—but what position will send you into wild, orgasmic bliss? You choose, and oh, the fun you will have deciding which position(s) work best for the both of you. On your first night together, don't obsess about your body. Do what makes you feel your sexiest, where he can advance and retreat, drag or coax, move up and down, go and return left or right, withdraw and thrust infrequently or repeatedly until you both climax. Here are some tips so you can absorb his essence to your fill.

THE BEST SEXUAL POSITIONS TIPS

- For the courtesan, *seppun*, "the kiss," was used sparingly, all the more erotic for being least expected: Lie on your back, keeping your legs at a ninety-degree angle, with your lover lying beside you. Raise the leg nearest to him high enough to allow him to enter you from under your thigh. His leg should cross over your body so you can use your thigh to control the depth of his penetration—and surprise him with a sensual kiss on the lips.

- The geisha energized her love life by breaking boundaries and taboos. If the guest couldn't wait to reach her small upstairs room in the *okiya*, teahouse, she

would kneel at the staircase land-
ing, facing the stairs. Their bodies pressed together tightly, she
would hold on to the staircase for
support as he held her hips and
penetrated her from behind. Don't
confine yourselves to a rigid routine that never changes. Something
new will make his climax—and
yours—more intense. Do you have
a tight, sexy butt? Suggest the "rear
door entry."

Thigh High

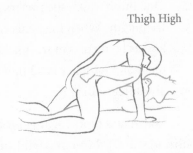

*Vary your lovemaking positions and experiment
to find those that please you and your partner*

- The games during a night's entertainment included pillow fights that often
  ended in intercourse. Add a pillow to enhance your sexual positions. The angle
  of his erection and your pelvis determine exactly what hot spots he will hit and
  how tightly he will feel gripped. Try a pillow under his cute butt while you're on
  top, or supporting your tailbone in the missionary position. Use pillows to prop
  yourself up when lying on a counter. Experiment with odd-size cushions for
  even more fun.

- Early courtesans were proud of their floor-length black hair and flaunted it by
  varying the "woman on top" position. Face his legs instead of his face and hold
  his feet for balance. He will love the great view of your sexy derrière and long
  hair. If his erection points out instead of up, this position will feel incredible to

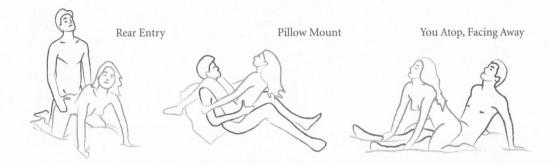

Rear Entry   Pillow Mount   You Atop, Facing Away

him. Be aware that a riding posture needs a stiff erection or you may bend him painfully if he inserts his penis too quickly and you go into action too fast.

- Sit astride facing him, his penis fully inserted. Lie back with your head and trunk between his wide-open legs, clasp his hands and begin slow, coordinated bucking movements to keep *him* erect and *you* close to orgasm for a long period of time.

- Try a standing position with you doing a handstand. He holds onto your buttocks with one hand while he inserts his penis into your vagina with the other. Not being able to see what he's doing as he moves inside you can be very sexy. This position provides deep penetration and works best if you have acrobatic abilities and can withstand pressure in your head.

- With your lover standing behind you and you bending over and resting on your palms, arch your back like a bridge in a Japanese garden as he grasps your hips and enters you from behind with slow, steady movements for deep penetration.

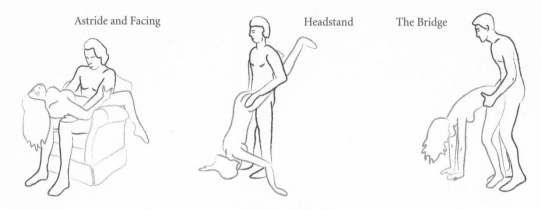

Astride and Facing   Headstand   The Bridge

Or, lie down and face him with one of your legs between his, and one of his between yours. Arch your back in this position for extra clitoral pressure from his thigh if he presses hard with it.

- Try this position favored by the courtesan to heighten her own sexual satisfaction: Both lie on your backs, with you on top. You will feel deep penetration when you arch away from him, making it easy for him to stimulate your breasts and clitoris. You can stay parallel to each another or "cross" over one another at a ninety-degree angle.

- When a geisha met secretly with her lover, they often made love in total darkness, relying only on their sense of touch to reach sexual satisfaction. Have your lover lie flat on his back with his legs spread, allowing you to lower yourself onto his penis, facing him. Lean backward with your legs at his sides and your toes pointing toward his head with both of you looking upward. Unable to see each other or move around, you focus more attention on each other's genitals.

You Atop, Facing Up

Face to Face in the Dark

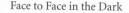

The Float

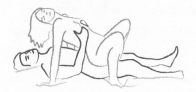

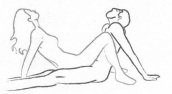

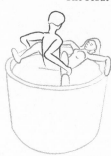

- The early bath attendants, *yuna*, engaged in sexual intercourse in unoccupied sections of public baths. A girl would lie on her back afloat while the man straddled her legs and penetrated her. Try this if you have a pool or Jacuzzi.

- Live sex sideshows in Old Edo featured a prostitute and a man performing unusual positions like this one: Rest your elbows on a chair and allow him to enter you, then wrap your legs around him as he lifts you up and holds you around the waist. Hold onto the chair as if doing a handstand while he thrusts in you.

To prolong their pleasure, Yoshiwara courtesans encouraged lovers to follow ancient Chinese Taoist mind-body techniques, whereby the man trained himself to delay or avoid ejaculation during lovemaking. With unhurried, shallow thrustings, deep breathing, slowing down or complete withdrawal when sensations reached a climatic point, and, at times, putting on the brakes with pressure on certain sex points, he controlled his sexual prowess. It was up to the courtesan to help him relax, since tension is the surest way to pre-

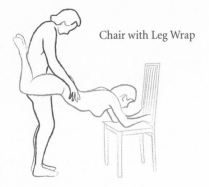

Chair with Leg Wrap

mature ejaculation. Prolong your pleasure, and his, by asking your lover to take his time.

Did he hit your G-spot? Not sure? Elusive, seductive, and incredibly sexy, your G-spot may be the one thing you are missing during sex.

YOUR G-SPOT

In *shunga,* when a courtesan was depicted lying back, feet on her lover's shoulders or on her belly as he penetrated her, her eyes closed in blissful abandon and lips parted in a sigh, it meant he had found her G-spot. So can your lover. Your G-spot is about the size of a quarter. It is located two or three inches inside your vagina, directly behind your pubic bone and clitoris. Your climax involves both clitoral and G-spot stimulation and is the most intense and pleasurable sensation you will experience. Here are some tips to help him.

Finding Your G-Spot Tips

- Have him insert his middle and index fingers about two inches inside your vagina. With the padded sides of his fingers facing the front wall of your canal, ask him to massage until he finds the spot, which may protrude slightly upon stimulation. He will know by the rapturous look on your face. Ask him to press lightly and with a rhythm you are comfortable with. Ready for more? Ask him to push down on your pubic mound to increase pressure on your G-spot.

- Intensify your orgasm: Ride astride and lean forward slightly. When you are about to climax, press into your pubic mound with three fingers. If you don't feel anything, press a few inches higher or lower until you do. Massage the area, using a firm circular motion to feel G-spot stimulation from the inside and the outside.

- For triple action fun, use your other hand to stimulate your clitoris while you rub your G-spot on the outside and his penis hits your G-spot inside. You will feel waves of excitement inside and outside your body—and your orgasm will last longer.

- Get on top facing away from him, his legs outstretched so together you form a "T" shape. As you move, lean forward as low as you can against his legs while still straddling his lap (hold his legs or ankles to keep your balance). Penetration from behind gives him better access to your G-spot and also a daring and naughty look at your *wareme-chan* thrusting on his penis. You're in control and he has a front row seat on the action.

- Lie on your side in an "L"-shaped position with your man lying on his side, his head toward your feet. As he enters you, stabilize yourself by placing your feet on his shoulders or neck. You will feel great penetration, not to mention G-spot contact.

Here you are, caught up in a tangled frenzy in your man's arms, his penis thrusting, you're swooning, your eyelashes fluttering—when are you going to have an orgasm? *When?*

"O" IS FOR ORGASM

In a *shunga* from a series entitled "Twelve Ways of Making Love" by Katsukawa Shuncho, circa 1785, the courtesan cries out to her lover as she experiences an orgasm, "Push deeper now! That's it, that's it . . . Oh! You're killing me again!"[35]

Such images were typical, but no artist portrayed a woman in orgasmic bliss better than the early-nineteenth-century master Katsushika Hokusai. Imagine a naked woman lying on rocks covered with green seaweed, in a rapturous swoon as an immense octopus feasts upon her vulva, while a small octopus hungrily nibbles at her mouth, its tentacle encircling her breast. This outrageously sensual depiction is the epitome of a woman in the exhaustive depths of orgasm. Reaching orgasm can be at once mysterious, wonderful, frustrating, and exhilarating—and, at times, elusive. If you're feeling sexy and in need of physical release, act on your feelings. Although it feels naughty, a quickie with that special someone can help your relationship. Meet him for lunch and do it in the back of his car, or make love on the living room floor—any place or time that deviates from your normal lovemaking routine. It takes the place of having an affair, giving you the illicit rush you get from doing something only "bad" girls do.

ORGASM TIPS

- You can attain a vaginal orgasm of maximum enjoyment during lovemaking with pubic squeeze motions: Tense your buttocks, press your thighs inward, and make a conscious effort to contract, then relax the vaginal muscles.

- Use breathing to control and intensify your orgasm. As you exhale, imagine you're pushing delicious sensations throughout your body instead of letting them build up below your waist. When you finally let go, you will feel the orgasm from head to toe.

- In an erotic poem a famous *oiran* wrote, " . . . I feel his *bonze* ["monk"] head straining against my chrysanthemum, then the scalding of his fire juice in my bowels."[36] Boost your orgasm by introducing him to the bit of skin between your anus and your vagina. The perineum is a nerve-packed point that produces electrifying sensations when he massages the area with his fingers.

- The *yujo,* or licensed prostitute, was known for her "cry in the night," *yonaki,* when she was having a great orgasm. Don't be embarrassed to make known your feelings when you're sexually excited. Laugh, shout, sing. Ask him to gag you if that turns you on, or stuff your hair in your mouth (a favorite of courtesans in *shunga*). The more you express pleasure, the more you exude sexual confidence, making you irresistible.

- The courtesan knew when her customer was about to climax because he would yell out, asking her where he should ejaculate. You both will experience orgasm in a new and exciting way if you sustain eye contact throughout your climaxes.

- The courtesan secretly enjoyed being known as an *otoko masari*, a woman who excels over a man,[37] including orgasm. His lasts about ten seconds and it *is* possible for him to have one without ejaculating. Some men are ready for another erection right away, but most need to wait at least twenty minutes. You don't. You possess the ability to have multiple orgasms. Experiencing *only* clitoral orgasms is okay. What makes you feel good is right for you.

The Courtesan's Sexual Positions

To perfect the art of her profession, the courtesan of Old Edo looked to guidebooks for new ways to please her lover. Among her favorites were the sexual positions from *The Mystic Master of the Grotto* by Dong Xuan Zi:[d]

- *Dragons Twisting*: Lie on your back; bend your legs. Your man kneels within your thighs, his left hand pushing your feet forward until they are past your breasts. His right hand inserts his penis into your vagina.
- *Seagulls Soaring*: Your man stands near the edge of the bed and lifts your legs high. He inserts his penis into your vagina.
- *White Tiger Jumping*: You bend over and lower your face. Your man stands behind you, one hand holding your hip, his other hand holding you by the ankle. He inserts his penis into your vagina.
- *Wild Horses Leaping*: You lie on your back. Your man lifts your feet and puts them over his shoulders. He inserts his penis deeply into your vagina.
- *Rock Soaring over the Dark Sea*: You lie on your back. Your man puts your feet on his upper arms. He stretches his hands down to clasp your waist, then inserts his penis.
- *Fish Eye-to-Eye*: You lie down facing each other, sucking each other's lips and tongues. Raise one leg above his body while he spreads his legs slightly. With one hand supporting your upraised leg, he inserts his penis into your vagina.
- *Butterflies Fluttering*: He lies on his back, his legs extended. You sit astride him, facing his head, your feet on the floor. Use your hand to insert his hard penis into your vagina.
- *Humming Ape Embracing the Tree*: He sits with his legs extended while you straddle his thighs, embracing him. He uses one hand to hold your buttocks and the other to insert his penis in you.
- *Stepping Tigers*: You bend over in a crawling position with your buttocks up and your head down. The man kneels behind you, clasping your belly. He inserts his penis and fills you up as deeply as he can, advancing and retreating.

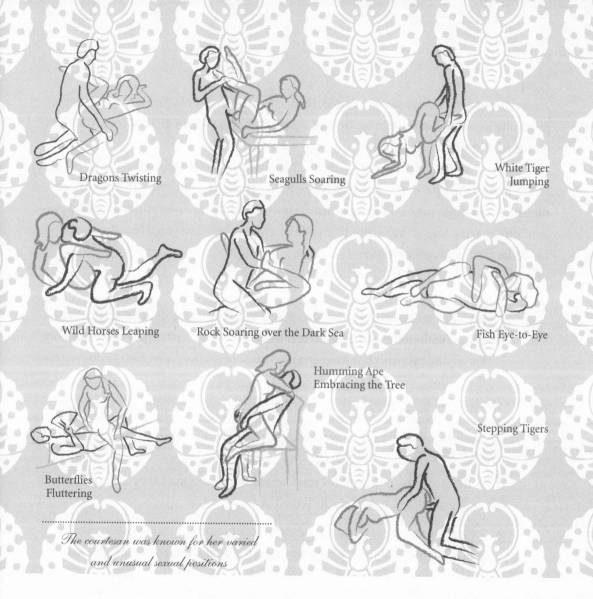

Dragons Twisting

Seagulls Soaring

White Tiger
Jumping

Wild Horses Leaping

Rock Soaring over the Dark Sea

Fish Eye-to-Eye

Humming Ape
Embracing the Tree

Stepping Tigers

Butterflies
Fluttering

*The courtesan was known for her varied
and unusual sexual positions*

POST SEX

A fantastic orgasm makes you exhausted, unable to move a muscle. You have, as a modern prostitute would say, *goru-in shita*, "scored a goal." You feel a warm glow of love. Your body is relaxed. But what is *he* feeling?

A *shunga* series titled *Komoncho*, "Notebook of Small Drawings," includes a pair of lovers after their passion is completely spent. She is smiling, her eyes half-closed; he leans under the mosquito net to fill a cup of tea.[38] How you and your lover prolong mutual pleasure after making love is important to creating harmony between you. Here are some tips for better post-sex togetherness.

Post-Sex Satisfaction Tips

- After he's made love to you, do as geisha and courtesans did and magically appear with hot, moist hand towels in a little wicker basket. These are not only for wiping his penis but soothing his heated brow. You want him to do it again, don't you?

- Tell him he was the greatest, whether he was or not. His ego can't support anything less. If he asks you, "How was it?" and you tell him anything but the best, there might not be a next time.

- You can also ask, "Where did you learn to do that?" Don't expect an answer, just a big grin. When he's ready, he'll do it again.

- Don't chatter on endlessly afterward, giving him tips on what you would like him to do the next time. This is the biggest mistake you can make. The last thing he wants to do is discuss a play-by-play of his performance with you.

• Once you've made love, don't assume that your commitment level has changed. Don't expect any more commitment *after* sex than before.

• *Your* orgasm may have made you more spiritually aware of yourself and the cosmos, but it is unlikely he has had the same feeling of enlightenment. It's not his nature.

Chapter 8

NAKED GAMES

Doing as if possessed by a deity and pulling out the nipples of her breasts, she pushed her skirt-string beneath her private parts. Then the Plain of High Heaven shook and the eight hundred myriad deities laughed together.

Kojiki, A.D. 712[1]

The kimono of the *tayu* was very long. To keep it from dragging, she would gather it up in one hand just beneath her magnificent, wide silk *obi*, allowing men a peek at her red under-slip. Later, in the privacy of her apartments under her patron's gaze, she would slowly undo her hair, letting it fall over her shoulders. Next, she would untie her *obi* and open her kimono to show him her beautifully embroidered silk undergarments. This simple act created excitement without frustration. He knew what was coming. When she opened her kimono, her posture revealed her as a woman of blood and fire, ready to satisfy his most sensual urges and erotic impulses. She intrigued him with unexpected beauty, then overwhelmed him with irresistible sensuality. She was also completely nude.

The *tayu was* both magic and sorcery, and symbolized life's most carnal pleasures. You also should revel in the enjoyment of your naked body. Celebrate your sexuality. Embrace it, show it, as if to say, *I have it, and it's a good thing.* Take responsibility for your sexual powers and use them to seduce him *and* pleasure yourself. But keep this in mind about games: Never do anything you don't want to do. Never do anything you consider demeaning. Never do anything unsafe.

STRIPTEASE

Western-style striptease was introduced to Japan after World War II during the U.S. Occupation (1945–52), when the girls chose to take off their clothes in theaters rather than turn to prostitution. The Japanese realized that nudity, something they regarded as natural, was much sought after by foreigners. So, instead of the Cherry Blossom Festival, they started the Festival of Breasts. A new word was coined, *nudo*, an idea that had not previously existed in Japan. *Sutorippu gekijo*, "striptease theaters" became popular.[2]

Stripping is every woman's overriding fantasy. It is both a defiant and seductive act, the classic test of your female sexual impact, where the art of the tease is your path to pleasure. Strippers look so incredible, powerful, and desirable. Incorporate the movements of the striptease into your workout and you will have the most amazing body in your life: strong and limber, taut and tight. A lean, feminine machine.

A striptease can be partial, simulated, decorated, even disguised. You are in complete control, deciding how much or how little you will remove. Never lose sight of that power and use it to your advantage. Do your dance slowly, have fun, and act like you own the place, including the man in it. You will, when your dance is over.

STRIPTEASE TIPS
- It all comes down to attitude. It doesn't matter what you take off, it's *how* you do it. Study strippers' routines in films or TV shows, then practice in front of a mirror until you feel confident enough to try it in front of him.

- Make sure your "stage" is set up and ready with the right lighting and décor.

- Check your music ahead of time and make certain it's cued in, then start the fireworks.

- Be in costume when he shows up at your door. You can either surprise him or find out ahead of time what turns him on. What you wear is important.

- Think of your outfit as layer upon interesting layer. Try a long dress that zips down far enough for you to give it your all. Make sure what you have on underneath is pretty and feminine, even sparkling. Years ago only professional strippers wore thongs; now you can buy them and other erotic underwear at fashion outlets.

- The courtesan wore high, high clogs. High heels elongate the leg to an erotic pinnacle. They are an absolute must and should never be removed during your strip.

- In geisha dances, movement was not as an end in itself, but a means to an end—a series of steps leading to striking a pose. Elevate the sexuality of your dance by striking a provocative pose when you feel the urge.

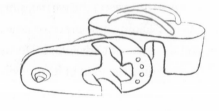

High geta or clogs slowed the gait of a courtesan and drew attention to her legs and feet

- Run your hands up and down

your curves, lingering on your breasts, hips, and thighs. Then unzip your gown and fling it aside. Keep him anticipating what you will do next. Stripping is more about *not* showing than about showing. That's why the dance is called "strip *tease.*"

- Take off your bra, shake your breasts, and pinch your nipples as you "bump and grind." You can either keep on or take off your G-string, then squat down on your haunches, looking at him with a sexy smile, letting him savor the proximity of your nakedness, making him sweat. If he reaches out to touch or pinch you, playfully smack his hand away, then run off, inviting him to follow . . . and make love to you.

- In Tokyo, a stripper never watches another stripper perform unless invited. Do not invite your girlfriends or his friends to watch you strip. Your strip is for you and your man *only*.

LAP DANCING

Seventeenth-century erotic novelist Ihara Saikaku noted that the ordinary women of the town often took as much pleasure in sex as their male counterparts, sometimes to the point of nymphomania.[3]

A steamy lap dance is a mutual pleasure. Slip into something that makes you feel sexy and feminine, whether it's lacy lingerie or a tight T-shirt and a thong. *And* high heels. Turn on your favorite music to loosen up your inhibitions. Poised over his lap and standing as close to him as you dare, move in time to the music, slowly tracing your body with your hands, up and down your breasts, circling your nipples, fanning them across your

How to Make Whipped Cream

- Heavy cream whips better than whipping cream due to its higher butterfat content. Light cream, also called coffee cream, does not whip.
- Before whipping, chill the cream, bowl, and beaters. Warm cream may not whip.
- An electric mixer works best. Begin at medium speed, moving the beater around in the bottom of the bowl to whip the cream evenly. As it thickens, reduce the speed so you can whip to fairly stiff peaks for spreading on his favorite parts of your anatomy.
- Add sugar and dry flavorings such as instant coffee, vanilla powder, or spices when you begin. Liquid flavorings such as vanilla or other extracts, brandies, or melted chocolate are best added at the end in small amounts so they won't soften the cream.
- Apply to your body promptly, since whipped cream does not retain its shape for long, unlike your man's penis as he licks it off.

pubic area. Then turn your back. Don't worry, he can't take his eyes off you. Bend over and run your fingers up the backs of your legs, all the way up to your tight buttocks. Trace your fingers down the crack and over your hips. Go for some grinding while you are doing your gyrations. Turn around and face him with a sexy, knowing smile. He knows what's coming next and he can't wait.

Biting seductively on your lower lip, push his knees apart and slither your body down the length of his torso. Remind him that he can look all he wants, but he can't touch until you tell him. You are in control. Let your hands roam all over your body, *everywhere*, testing where your sexual power comes from and where it will take you. Finish your seduction by simulating the sex act with him and see where it goes from there. There's no place for *him* to go but up.

HIS JUST DESSERTS

In Tokyo's red-light district of Kabukicho, a man can go to a club specializing in whipped cream and get his fill of the creamy stuff. For a set fee, he takes a girl to a private room, removes her clothes, and covers her in lactic love. If he is unable to lick her clean, he is fined.

Play this game with your man and *you* determine what the fine will be. A night of seduction with whipped cream is enticing. You can use ready-made, but the best is from your own recipe. Whipped cream is fast to prepare. Make it ahead of time to get it perfect and have ready. His performance with his tongue has a lot to do with the smoothness of the cream. He won't be able to get enough of it *or* you.

You've stripped down to nothing or close to it, had your fill of whipped cream. What's next? Making love? No, keep the momentum going—and his anticipation level high—with your own private live sex show.

LIVE SEX SHOWS

In Old Edo's Yoshiwara, the courtesan was the pinnacle entertainer. Her performances were exclusive, for her patron's eyes alone. Beyond her private rooms lay a vibrant, raucous world of sex. A common sight was a *yujo* on a theater stage, singing a vulgar song as she gradually undid her *obi* and opened her kimono, revealing herself to ogling onlookers.[4] Until after the Meiji period, *misemono*, the sideshows popular at fairs and festivals, included among their acts a girl hoisting her kimono as men blew between her parted thighs with a feathered tickler.[5] Other shows were evocative, daring, and bizarre in tone. Men with exceptionally long penises and women with extravagant pubic hair were featured. The open display of intercourse between a stallion and a woman was recorded from the 1790s up to 1863, but the practice came to an end when a woman passer-by was killed.[6]

In 1958, Japan passed the Entertainment Control Law designed to limit the influence of the *yakuza*, Japanese mafia, in the *mizushobai*, or sex trade.[7] Yet in Tokyo's Kabukicho district, and its counterpart in Osaka, a fast and loose reputation of nearly three centuries is flourishing. Live sex shows thrive. Beginning mid-morning and finishing before midnight, women dance naked and perform sexual intercourse on stage for the admission price. Most theaters feature a small, circular additional stage, which rotates when the action heats up. Some girls become "idol strippers," *aidoru sutorippa,* receiving fan mail and becoming the focus of magazine stories.[8] The *himo*, pimp, is involved, but he is considered no different from a manager in other businesses.[9] This world of sex exists in a parallel universe alongside the ordinary world, never touching it.

Although the bondage, sadomasochism, lesbian acts, and audience participation in modern sex shows can be raw and at times shocking, the provocative techniques and moves of the girls are instructional if you have the daring. "Pretend" can be arousing for both of you. Here are some tips if you want to give him his own private live sex show.

LIVE SEX SHOW TIPS

- In Tokyo, high-class intimate bars with no stage often have private shows. Showcase your act impromptu in an open space in your living room, a cozy nook, sunken conversation pit, or a polished tiled entryway.

- In *open steji,* "open stage," a girl squats or lies inches from onlookers, spreading her thighs as far as possible. A pink spotlight highlights her delicate flesh. Lie on your back and open your legs, gracefully tracing an arc in the air like an opening fan. A big flashlight or a penlight and a magnifying glass will give your partner a better view. Don't let the light get too close to your body. Things will be hot enough.

- Squatting over sheets of paper, girls write messages of good luck with writing brushes gripped in their vaginas. Try it. Your writing may not the best, but he's certain to keep this note in a special place. The girls also dab their genitals with black ink; audience members then press white paper to make personalized "fish" prints. You don't have to worry about your writing with this one.

- In "vinyl clubs," a girl is wrapped in a vinyl bag. Men feel her breasts and genitals through the vinyl, never touching her skin. To heighten foreplay, wrap yourself up in a sensual fabric and let him touch *you* through the material.

- Inviting a man on stage, the girl removes his pants and folds his underwear, allowing him to keep on his shirt and necktie. Next, she swabs his penis with alcohol and puts on a condom. He fondles and suckles her, has intercourse with her, then returns to his seat. Follow the same scenario for a stimulating twist on making love.

- *Tachi sho,* "touch show," is where men take turns fondling girls. For "customer service," a girl approaches the audience with a small basket containing a Polaroid camera and a tub of wet-wipes. After the men clean their hands, they are invited to feel her body and take do-it-yourself porn shots. Charge up your digital camera and let him take his best shot, then check out the photos on your computer.

A sex show is high stakes foreplay. You have turned him on to the point where he can't wait to make love to you. Up the ante with a little game or two first.

SEX GAMES

In an Old Edo legend, a monk turned ferryman with an indefatigable penis fell prey to the appetites of the lady of a castle and her three maids. The women kept him prisoner, inventing games to play, including shutting him up in a large bag, " . . . having first cut a hole big enough for his penis to protrude when required."[10] A sex game is *any* game that gives you and your partner pleasure. Here are some ideas to get you started.

> *SEX GAME TIPS*
>
> - At *nopan kissa* (a contraction of "no-panty *kissaten* [tea shop]"),[11] waitresses wear nothing but a little apron and serve expensive cups of tea and coffee on mirrored tables above mirrored floors. Try this at home, placing small mirrors at strategic angles, or give your lover a hand mirror so he can see your best side.
>
> - Make your hairdryer into a wind machine by attaching a few feathers to the nozzle with strong thread. Sweep them over each other's palms or soles of the feet, or other areas if he is game, or your breasts, belly, and between your thighs. Never use the hot air button or strong air. Never blow into your vagina or any other body orifice.
>
> - Some hostess bars feature a game with regulars called "strip dice," where everyone ends up nude. The final throw takes place in a hotel room. Play this one with loaded dice. He won't care if you win.
>
> - Another hostess bar game is "pluck it." Men and girls alternate throwing the die. Each throw must beat the one before it. Whoever fails must give up a pubic hair.

The successful thrower plucks the loser. You can improve on this sexy game: The winner plucks the pubic hair of the loser with his or her teeth.

- The *yujo* took pride in her plucked and clipped pudendum, indicating her sexual skills.[12] If your man is turned on by bare genitals, let him shave you. With both of you nude, stand with one leg on the closed toilet seat while he sits on the edge of the tub. Use a sharp, but not too sharp, razor, and soap. He'll get an erection, and as he feels your vagina, you can both enjoy your juices beading up on the naked lips like dew on the pink petals of a cherry blossom.

The ultimate sex game requires not only complete trust and confidence in your lover, but silken ropes and pretty knots. Bondage. Taboo, or "to do"? You won't know until you ask.

SHIBARI: "EROTIC BONDAGE"

The Japanese have turned knot tying into a beautiful art, from gift packaging to the *obijime*, cord, encircling a geisha's sash. *Shibari,* bondage, began with the martial art of restraint known as *hojojutsu,* in which samurai practiced capturing or detaining the enemy with ropes in the least possible amount of time. Hemp rope, *asanawa,* became a symbol of power.

Shibari is one of the most popular themes in *shunga*: a prostitute is shown stripped to the waist and tied to a rafter as punishment; a nude girl is bound with intricate knots; or a courtesan is tied spread-eagled to a pole and gagged with her own hair, eyes wide, head lolling back and toes arched upward in ecstasy as a man penetrates her. Since the 1960s, special theaters have featured a *nawashi*, rope artist,[13] to tie up a *dorei,* a willing female.[14] Today, erotic bondage figures prominently in *manga* and porn videos.

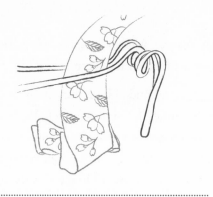

Indulge in elegant bondage with a decorative obi or sash and a length of Japanese cord

No longer the taboo it once was in America, bondage is the second most popular fantasy after group sex. It is resistance training of a sexual kind, a symbolic domination rather than physical or mental. When you are tied up à la *nawa-kesho,* "applying rope like a cosmetic art,"[15] you look and feel sexy because it builds anticipation of what is to come—you! This heightens your arousal.

When you're tied up and ready to go, he can kiss, tickle, fondle, masturbate, or tease you to orgasm. While unable to move, a slow orgasm, *oruganzumi,*[16] can be a mind-blowing experience if you are willing to let it happen. Let go and yell as loud as you want, reveling in your pleasure and loving every moment. When it is his turn, fasten his hands, blindfold him, and seduce him by stroking his penis until he is fully aroused. Then stop. Then more. Make it different each time. Not knowing what comes next will drive him wild to the point where he is begging to be untied. And when you do, he will return the pleasure of delicious torture so you can reach orgasm in each other's arms. Bondage is liberating. Is that a surprise?

Shibari Tips
- Bondage kits are available for what aficionados call a "pleasurable lashing," but don't scare him off by greeting him in a black leather miniskirt, six-inch heels, and cracking your whip.

- Genuine *shibari* requires rope. In general, you can use leather or rubber straps, silk cords, pajama belts, bathrobe sashes, scarves, or ribbons. You want the knot to be comfortable but firm, so it can't be gotten out of easily. Be careful with stockings. They can be difficult to untie quickly should an emergency come up.

- Take turns. You want equality of pleasure, don't you?

- Who goes first? If you enjoy allowing him to be the *meijin*, "skilled master," spread your arms and legs like the courtesans in *shunga* and go for it. You want him to bring you to orgasm without feeling uncomfortable or getting loose, while you struggle as hard as you like.

- Tying him up can be interesting, especially if he is the "alpha male" type. With you as the *onna shujin*, "mistress," he can relax without worrying about his performance.

- *Shunga* often depict a courtesan tied to a post on the ground. Your four-poster bed will work, or a soft futon on the floor with your hands and feet tied to something nearby that can withstand you pulling hard on it.

- Or, have him tie your wrists, ankles, elbows, soles, thumbs, and big toes together. These are "sex points," where compression boosts arousal. Another fun "rope trick" is *shinju*, "pearls," tying up your breasts to emphasize your nipples. For extra fun, try *sakuranbo*, "cherry," tying up your buttocks to emphasize your vagina.

- Velvet-lined handcuffs can be exciting and don't hurt like metal ones, but neither cuffs nor chains give compression. Any apparatus that locks can pose frustration if it doesn't work properly, not to mention danger or embarrassment if it won't come off.

- Gagging is optional. Avoid using adhesive on your mouth. It will do more than ruin your lipstick and is difficult to remove.

- Blindfolds are a matter of trust. Silk blindfolds build a titillating sense of suspense. Silk's sensual feel will enhance your experience and what you can't see will thrill you.

- Private sex shows sometimes include participants stripping and playfully whipping each other. Don't be afraid to tell him how far he can go. You can always be open to negotiations. No action should ever be painful or dangerous.

- Try playing headmistress to his naughty schoolboy. Take charge with a pocket paddle that delivers varying sensations ranging from a tickle to a stinging feeling.

- Or reverse the power play and be his slave as he wields a stretchy, versatile latex whip. You will sweat as well as experience a delicious orgasm as the foot-long elastic strands gently create a beguiling blush on your breasts or quivering buttocks.

- For a different kind of adventure that will drive you over the edge, experiment with nipple clips that tease with pressure from adjustable clamps attached to a battery pack. You or your man can set them tingling with vibrations focused right where they provide the greatest sensation.

Some Basic Bondage Rules

Words of caution: Do not try bondage unless you have complete confidence in your partner. Discuss what you mean by being dominated, along with his ideas. Only begin with mutual consent. It is imperative to discuss signals beforehand; neither of you should ever be in a position where you are incapable of signaling. Let him know how he can distinguish any distress, from physical, such as cramped wrists or legs, or pain anywhere in your body, to sexual. Never tie anything around the neck. Nothing must be inserted in the mouth that can block an air passageway. All gags and knots must be quick-release. Never leave the room when he is tied up and helpless, and demand the same from him. Don't keep him or allow yourself to be tied up for more than half an hour. Avoid group bondage scenarios with his friends or strangers. Someone could be careless, or worse, put you in a dangerous and life-threatening position. Trust is everything.

You might not be adept at bondage games right away. Your knots can come apart at an inopportune moment, or you can't get them undone, or you climax quicker than you thought you would. It's all part of the game.

ENTERTAINING THE PEEPING TOM

In Japan, voyeurism has long been a popular pastime, a titillating theme of *shunga* where even mice sometimes join in the fun, and a favorite in erotic literature. *The Story of an Incorrigible Libertine Who Was Small Enough to Fit into a Pocket,* published anonymously in 1711, tells the tale of a man given a pill by a faerie that made him so small he could slip unnoticed into others' amorous encounters.[17]

In real life, the curious of Old Edo used telescopes to spy on lusty neighbors. In their own homes, men and women were known to peep around the easily moved room-dividing screens. In crowded city streets, spectators of *both* sexes ogled fast-moving young porters on errands, their kimonos rolled up to the groin. If you want to add some excitement to your lovemaking, do as the geisha did when she allowed the *maiko* to peek from behind the screen to learn about sex. Be naughty the next time you and your man fool around and leave your shades open.

Today, clubs feature small cubicles with one-way mirrors, where customers peer into a "bedroom" and watch a nude girl play with her breasts, rub her genitals against a door handle, masturbate with cucumbers and bananas, then take a shower. Or, the girl masturbates on a couch behind a plate glass window while exchanging sexual banter on the telephone with her customer. On stage, girls walk back and forth offering themselves for foreplay. Men proffer their fingers, which the girls swab and sheath in plastic gloves and then allow to be inserted into their vaginas.

PLAYFUL MASTURBATION TIPS

- The courtesan enjoyed elaborate finger-stimulation by her lover, including his thumb in her anus and his fingers and tongue in her vagina. She also used vegetables like radishes, mushrooms, and carrots to achieve orgasm. Never downplay the enjoyment you can receive from non-penis penetration.

- Set up your own peep show if your man is daring. He can stand outside your window (no nosy neighbors, please) and watch you masturbate as you talk to him on your cell phone.

- In a dimly lit "pink salon," a young Japanese prostitute allows a customer to fondle her. Then she uses manual skills to bring him to orgasm. This game is best tried at home. If you're feeling very wild, try a dark corner of a club or restaurant, but use discretion.

- Men find a masturbating woman fascinating and mysterious. Just *hearing* you talk about it can be a turn-on. So, show him the real thing. Put on something sexy and revealing. Try a pair of split panties or slowly take off your panties as he watches. Flick your fingers lightly over your belly to your pubic area, teasing him by circling your pleasure spot rather than putting them inside. When he—and you—can't stand it any longer, insert them and stimulate your clitoris. For maximum enjoyment focus on the shaft, not the small bean. Go ahead and moan. It's a turn-on to both of you.

- If he agrees, tie him up and make him watch you masturbate to orgasm. Start with your panties on, fondling yourself through the silky fabric until you feel comfortable with pulling them down. Your gyrations will make him crazy and his struggling will turn *you* on. After you climax, you can untie him and . . . what you do next is up to you.

SEX TOYS

Rain beat down on the blue-tiled roof of the geisha teahouse as raw, hungry sighs of pleasure echoed throughout the rooms. Male and female. Female and female. The clink of metal balls hitting each other and the crunch of a dried leather "mushroom" sliding into a moist pink vagina mixed with the soft patter of rain. In the nineteenth century, one firm, Yotsume-ya, operated sex shops selling artificial penises and vulvas, aphrodisiacs, pastes for pederasts, and love potions to courtesans.[18] Erection aids, masturbation devices, clitoral stimulators, lubricants, contraceptives, books and prints for instruction, and hygienic tissues were also available.

In the erotic world of sex toys, you can revitalize your life force with dildos, metal balls, and love beads. Sex toys can be fun, funky, and give you a fantastic orgasm. They are the symbolic linking of your female passion and power with his penis, the ultimate "sex toy." Use these devices in your art of seduction. Why should you, you ask, when you have the real thing? Sex toys encourage your imagination to explore a world different from everyday reality. They bring alive the sensual spirit dwelling within you both. As a geisha once wrote in her diary, "I kissed her and noticed a *harigata* in her hand. I took it eagerly. Who knows where this journey will end?"[19]

Whatever your need or desire, there is a sex toy for you. If you're questioning how he will feel when confronted with a toy that resembles a longer, wider version of his genitalia, chances are he isn't intimidated. More than likely, he likes it. Ask him.

You are capable of enjoying multiple orgasms and feeling endless waves of pleasure. If your man is sure of himself and filled with confidence, he will encourage you to use sex toys. He can't vibrate his tongue, penis, or fingers at a constant high speed, so he's grateful for the help. Always let him know that sex toy play is one kind of pleasure, but it's *not* the ultimate pleasure. Playing with love beads or a dildo is merely a warm-up to the main act. Ready?

DILDOS

A geisha without a lover, unable to enjoy the scent of the loincloth, was referred to as "dried fish." Yet, she had a most pleasurable way to satisfy her needs: her *harigata*, dildo, an artificial penis usually made of leather, and at times a strap-on made from horn or ivory.[20] Inserting it into her vagina, she lay back and let it work its magic. The young *yujo*, as her initiation into *toko no higi*, "bedroom manners," was instructed with the aid of a dildo on

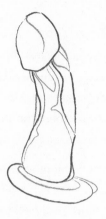

how to pleasure a man, as well as how to make him climax quickly and how to fake a convincing orgasm.

Dildos may be used vaginally or anally and typically don't vibrate as they titillate your erotic zone. Here is a guide to dildos to help you choose the perfect one for you.

Many old Japanese harigata, or dildos, are made of polished, artistically carved wood

Dildo Tips

- The *harigata* was carved or molded to look like a real penis. You can get a dildo with a smooth surface; those made of silicone are easy-to-clean, firm, and warm to your body temperature. Or, if you want a toy that looks and feels like the real thing, choose cyberskin. Some dildos feature a convenient flat base and are available in your choice of skin tones, with or without pubic hair.

- Like the penis in *shunga,* the *harigata*'s size was often exaggerated. The average modern dildo is long and slim, 6 to 7 inches by 1¼ to 1½ inches, a good choice for solo play that will give deep penetration. If long dildos bump your cervix (it will hurt), get a shorter model. A unique style features a flexible spine in the shaft, allowing you to mold the toy into any shape you like. Try doing that with *his* hard-on.

- Geisha often used a *kotori,* "little bird," a harness and rope suspension,[21] with a dildo of leather, buffalo horn, or tortoiseshell.[22] Strapped to her heel, the dildo gave solitary pleasure when she sat down upon it, her ankle held up by a sling around her neck to give a better swing to the sensual movement. Modern harnesses, with two waist straps and two leg straps that each snap onto the dildo ring, allow you to individualize the fit. They give greater penetration if you are on the receiving end, or, for an entirely new experience, can put you in control.

- Old Edo sex manuals recommended the *ryochi-dori*, "dual plover," or double dildo.[23] It was used by the courtesan and the bonze for the extra penis needed in threesomes. You also can make use of the double dildo. Designed to fit two bodies comfortably during simultaneous penetration, one end is short and curved, the other longer and straighter. If you are wearing the harness, insert the short end into your vagina first, then penetrate your partner either vaginally or anally with the longer end.

- In the 1800s, small inns providing food, lodging, and entertainment popped up around Tokyo's Shinjuku railroad station.[24] Today it's a red-light district, where a stripper might offer a dildo to a man in the audience, who then pushes it deep inside her vagina. She takes it out and offers it to the next man. Incorporate this into your striptease if it's right for you.

VIBRATORS

According to folklore, the courtesan underwent rigorous training for her first night of sexual intercourse. Like the prostitutes who came after her, she was taught to pull an egg into her vagina, then break it when given the signal.[25] This made her vaginal muscles strong so she could grip a penis tightly. Vibrators with an egg-shaped "pink rotor" have replaced real eggs. It is connected to a multispeed power pack; you turn it on and off and adjust the speed with your thumb for more buzz if your honey is tired.

The newest vibrators are light in weight, noiseless, self-contained, and oscillating. They offer pleasure and a way to experiment and control your orgasm by manipulating both your clitoris and vagina. Some can reach your sometimes-elusive G-spot. Some have unique features for compelling and sensual stimulation. What is right for you? It depends on what makes you feel good. If you're like most women, you probably reach orgasm primarily from clitoral stimulation, as your clitoris is highly responsive to vibration. If you like a focused touch, look for a vibrator with a smaller tip; if you don't like direct stimulation, try one with a bigger head that will elongate your sensations. A vibrator allows you to experience longer, stronger stimulation that can take you over the top.

Vibrator Tips

- Try a small, animal shaped model on a wire connected to a control box. Its many protrusions (ears, eyes, and tail) tease and tickle with different vibrations. Cute types include rabbits and ones with fox ears.

- Or, cuddle the "puppy" against your vulva so its tongue licks your clitoris.

- Try Mr. Pink, a "swinging" version that moves from side to side as it vibrates. It is designed with the smaller vaginas of Japanese women in mind.

- For discretion away from home, try a lipstick-shaped vibrator. Less than three inches long, it fits into your purse or pocket.

- For sensuous, private underwater pleasures, Japanese women love the I Rub My Duckie vibrator. Press the specially designed switch hidden in its back and it undulates, giving internal and external stimulation.

- Experiment with vibrators made for other purposes. The Kitty massager (resembling a famous children's mascot) is very popular in Japan. Its battery-operated stick, made for massaging the neck and shoulders, delivers strong vibration through the Kitty's extra-large head. Another popular vibrator is the *Vibrating Ecstasy Brush*: The soft head is ribbed for extra pleasure: a "tickling brush" on the other end can be used wherever it feels good.

- Share the pleasure of your vibrator with your partner while having sex. The versatile ring-style "clit stimulator" has bumps facing out. Worn around the base of his shaft, it also serves as a penis ring reminiscent of those used by the courtesans of Old Edo.

- A unique Japanese vibrator called Kuri Kuri, "chestnut" (resembling your clitoris), can be used by both of you. He slips the unit over his penis, then enters you. The pressure of his body against yours makes it turn on. Or, ask him to buzz it against your clitoris, or tell him to sit back and watch you handle it. He will be turned on just by seeing *you* turned on.

- For more fun, try a remote control vibrator. You wear the slender unit discreetly under your clothes, then hand the remote to him. When you see a sexy smile from across the room, you'll know he is about to turn you on with the flick of a switch.

RIN NO TAMA

The geisha is known for her secret smile as she sits upon her heels, gently swaying back and forth. It could be she is enjoying the pleasure of metal balls inserted into her vagina, so that any movement of her body produces a gentle and persistent vibration. *Rin no tama* balls made their way into Japan in the late fifteenth century and originally were made of silver. One ball contains a blob of mercury and the other a tiny tongue of copper. The balls vibrate even on the palm of your hand, and it is claimed they emit a tiny sound like a high-pitched tuning fork.[26]

      The modern versions, called *benwa* balls, are usually three-quarters of an inch in diameter. They are made from a variety of substances, including gold plate, silver, steel, plastic, Lucite, and any combination. You insert them, and as you sway to and fro, the vibrations as they knock together send a range of sensations throughout your body, from pleasurable to ecstatic. You can use *benwa* balls safely, either vaginally or anally. The best part is you can use them quietly wherever you are, giving *you* the geisha's secret smile.

Erotic Ball Tips

- A man can also enjoy these *benwa* balls when you insert them before making love. They tickle the top of his penis when he is inside you. They are said to increase his potency.

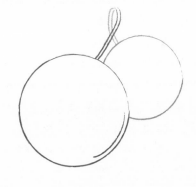

Erotic sex toys can be sphere-shaped and held together with cord for easy removal

- Legend has it there is a link between the oyster and your vagina because each contains a "pearl." "Pearls," vaginal or anal love beads, offer a range of climaxes. Insert the string of beads, then pull them out slowly or quickly depending upon the orgasm you desire. This is one time you can let him pull your strings.

- A different, slightly larger toy consists of two ball bearings each encased in a larger plastic sphere covered with silicone. The spheres are joined together with a piece of nylon cord for easy retrieval from your vagina after use.

- The Cherry Bomb vibrator is another version. Shaped like two cherries sharing the same stem, these pink and yellow balls give pleasure with two different and distinct vibrating patterns. The "cherries" are attached to a cord leading to a flat control panel that allows you to control the speed of the globes.

Nuguishi is the crumpled paper seen strewn around the exhausted lovers in *shunga*, indicating that lovemaking has taken place.[27] Cleanliness is important to your art of seduction. Be wary of contracting a urinary tract infection when using a sex toy or during intercourse. Never clean a toy with rubbing alcohol. It will eat away at the surface and make it painful as well as dangerous to use the next time. Because the hard, non-porous substances of *benwa* balls don't absorb bacteria, you can use them longer than other sex toys, except one: his penis. It comes with a lifetime guarantee.

You have your favorite sex toy, but what about him?

PENILE AIDS

The *yujo* was known for her unusual sexual skills. She would fit dried rings of sea slug over his penis or a *higozuiki*, a ring or thong tightly bound around the penile shaft.[28] These devices encouraged and maintained a hard erection by temporarily interrupting the return blood supply. This not only made him stiff, it also made him rough for *her* more pleasurable sensation.

PENILE AIDS TIPS

- Wrap a hair scrunchie around the base of your lover's testicles and penis after he's fully erect. (Use a macho color; he won't let you do it if it's pink.) Wrap it twice if it's loose. The scrunchie should be snug, but not so tight it's uncomfortable.

- After he's "scrunched up," kiss or stroke his penis lovingly. Don't be surprised if he moans more than usual. That extra squeeze you have given him at the base of his genitals keeps the blood trapped inside his erection and gives him undeniable pleasure.

- Edo-era courtesans offered their lovers a range of other pleasure-giving devices like a *kabutogata,* glans-cap of hard material, or a *dogata,* penile-shaft tube, some latticed (*yoroigata*) or with a glans-cap (*yasogata*).[29] You can find similar items for your man on adult-oriented websites and in specialty stores.

- Pearls, believed to increase potency when one or more are surgically inserted under the skin and down the length of his penis, will also increase your enjoyment when he penetrates you.

ARTIFICIAL VAGINAS

In the sex shops of nineteenth-century Japan, a man could choose from a wide variety of artificial vulvas for his pleasure, everything from an expensive replica of a young girl's, accurate in every way, to a " . . . carved cantaloupe melon cunningly inserted into his bed roll."[30] If you are curious how his penis looks penetrating your love box, try an artificial vagina for a new point of view.

ARTIFICIAL VAGINA TIPS

- If you or your partner desires an artificial vagina, try a warm-water model. The skin-like texture creates realistic sensations. He can ejaculate into a removable, washable, lubricated latex "packet" surrounded by the walls of the bladder.

- A foam-rubber type offers a different experience. The clasping sensation upon his penis, simulating the contractions of your vagina, is heightened by an air bladder inflated by a bulb at the end of the rubber tubing.

LIFE-SIZE SEX DOLLS

The floating world of seventeenth-century Japan prided itself on its devotion to revelry and pleasure, and on the exquisite beauty of the courtesans. If a gentleman was unable to procure the favors of an *oiran*, he could acquire a *ukiyo ningyo*, an erotic doll, to indulge his most sensual sexual needs.[31]

If your man is interested in a threesome with you and a life-size sex doll, don't worry. It's a fun way to enjoy a threesome without worrying about him falling for the other woman. She may have bigger breasts and a flat belly, but she can't whisper words of love in

Silly and Fun Sex Toys

Playing naked games is more than taking off your clothes. It's what you play with and how you do it. Here are some fun accessories to make your foreplay "for play."

- Use an "erect penis" bottle stopper to keep the champagne bubbly while you pop his cork.

- Put on a pair of classic penis-nose glasses or mammary-nose glasses when he comes to pick you for a date and watch *his* eyes bug out.

- Flaunt your clitoris by wearing butterfly crotchless panties with a pearl and sequin detail on the front.

- Reach for scratch 'n' sniff thongs in rose, cherry, peppermint, or tropical. He won't be able to get enough, whether you are wearing them or not. The scent may last for several washings but its effects last a lot longer.

- Get him "glow in the dark" boxer shorts. Imagine turning off the lights and seeing his penis slowly rising through them.

- Try teasing his penis with a foot-long ostrich feather. It feels exquisitely soft and ticklish when trailed across his skin.

- You can use suction for pleasure in your clitoris, *kuri-chan*. Known as Kuri-Cap, the set of two latex caps fits over your clitoris and stays attached by suction. These soft rubber bulbs (large and small caps) will stick to any part of your body.

- Stimulate your clitoris with special creams that, when rubbed into the underside of your love bean, are supposed to increase the blood flow to that region. You can intensify your sensitivity with a delightful tingling sensation by using a cream with peppermint—and smell good, too. Some contain L-arginine, an amino acid that can result in the dilation of blood vessels when ingested. The effects have not been proven topically, but manufacturers claim they increase desire and orgasmic potential. For the perfect blend of spontaneity and orgasmic thrills, there is one accessory that always works: manual stimulation. Your hand or his. Or both.

his ear or stroke his penis. *Or* make him breakfast. Here are some tips to help you enjoy the sensuality of a life-size sex doll that will have you both in orgasmic bliss.

Sex Doll Tips

- In Japan, life-size dolls modeled after computer game characters are available. Approximately $4,000 buys a fully adjustable doll with fourteen points of articulation, including fingers and neck.[32] She comes with a biography listing her birthday, favorite hobby, likes and dislikes, and her blood type. (Blood type is popularly used in modern Japan to determine personality.)[33]

- The inflatable "love pillow" is a full-size, dual-sided re-creation of a popular Japanese actress. Just under five feet tall when inflated, it is made of durable thick, soft plastic and is fully functional with front and back genital openings.

- Your man can have a life-size doll custom made to specification from an extensive list of options, from body and head to fingernail color. Her ultra-flesh-like silicone skin has a pleasant, fruity fragrance. Her completely articulated stainless steel and aluminum skeleton allows for anatomically correct positioning, and she is always relaxed and ready. Her vulva and anal cavities are soft, slippery, and very elastic, snug enough to accommodate his penis and allow deep insertion, whatever his size. Her fingers can close and grip. The three of you can take a bath together. She can withstand over four hundred degrees of heat and is not hollow, so water can't become trapped inside. The price is approximately $6,000.

- She comes dressed in a mini-dress, bra, panties, thigh-high stockings, and high heels. Letting the doll wear your clothes should be *your* decision, not his.

- If he prefers, a lower torso is available. It begins right above the belly button, terminates at mid-thigh, and has vaginal and anal entries. It is available in all skin tones with choice of pubic hair. The price is considerably lower: $1,500.

- Like every female, the life-size sex doll needs maintenance. A silicone repair kit contains everything he needs to fix small tears, including tubes of high strength silicone adhesive and skin-colored silicone for cosmetic repairs.

- If you want to get him jealous, go for a foursome and order your own life-size male sex doll for approximately $7,000.[34]

Whether you tie each other up, play sexy games in a stage-like setting, strip for your lover, or masturbate together, the ultimate pleasure is the harmony of your bodies and souls. But what if you have those sexy urges away from home? Where can you go for "quickie" sex that's not only satisfying but fun? Try a love hotel.

LOVE HOTELS

The scene is your lunch hour. You're on your way to meet him. You wander through a crowded mall in the fast-paced confusion of shoppers, seeking a quiet spot—somewhere, anywhere—you can brush up against his crotch, grab his cute butt, and whisper naughty words in his ear. Where can you be alone with him where no one will see you? There *is* such a place in Japan. It's called a love hotel.

As far back as Old Edo, pilgrims looking for a night of pleasure stayed in *otebiki-jaya,* short-term lodging.[35] The love hotels so popular today developed out of a 1960s curfew barring women in men's hotel rooms after nine P.M. A businessman taking a bar hostess to a Western-style hotel would be embarrassed by the gazes and smirks of desk clerks and other couples who knew why they were there. The respectable businessman sought an alternative to satisfy his sexual urges. The love hotel was born.

Today a thriving industry of more than twenty thousand love hotels offers temporary anonymity in nearly every town. Most love hotels are located near big train stations and major highway exits, and in entertainment districts. Their well-advertised presence is undeniable evidence that extramarital affairs are commonplace, though the hotels have changed their name. The phrase *rabu hoteru*, "love hotel," is no longer used, although the abbreviation *rabu-ho* is still heard. The hotels prefer to be known as fashion hotels, couples hotels, boutique hotels, leisure hotels, or theme hotels, etc. A small number take reservations and most have member cards giving frequent users a discount. Discount coupons are common in popular dating magazines.

Providing complete privacy, secrecy, and charging by the hour instead of by the night, the love hotel encourages temporary romance. Some even provide girls with the rooms. A symbol above the hotel name discreetly advertises what goes on inside: the *sakasa-kurage*, "upside down jellyfish." A circle with three wispy lines above, it represents steam rising from a pool of water and is used on Japanese maps to indicate hot springs resorts. Since these resorts are where Japanese men go for sensual pleasures, love hotels that provided similar services adopted the same symbol. Signboards are usually well lit with colorful, neon *katakana* (Japanese phonetic letters) or the English word "Hotel" surrounded by twinkling stars. Sometimes overly large objects are mounted on the roof, e.g., a thirty-foot mock Statue of Liberty or the QE2. There are three prices: A "rest fee" for a stay from one to three hours; a more expensive overnight "stay," though you can't check in until nine or ten

P.M.; and "service" or "free time" during the day, when you can stay as long as you want for a fixed price.

Every service is discreet. Parking facilities are concealed underground. The garage attendant even provides a license plate cover. The lobby lacks doorman, furnishings, and front desk. Some have a "man behind the curtain" who communicates only through a little slit to exchange money and the key. Others are high-tech: a big panel displays pictures of the various rooms. Some are lighted, indicating they are available. A paper card with the chosen room number or the room key drops out. A trail of flickering floor lights leads to the nearest elevator. When lovemaking is over, room charges are automatically added up; the door is often locked until payment. Guests insert payment in a machine by the door or put the hotel card in the slot of the control panel and push the button, or return the key at a pay window in the lobby. They see no one and no one sees them.

Inside, a businessman and his secretary (often the case) leave office routine behind for a world of heart-shaped and rotating beds, gaudy lighting, pornographic videos, and if they pay extra, sumptuous food. Their room is equipped with a refrigerator, private karaoke, wide-screen TV, games console, sex toys, and luxury bathrooms with Jacuzzi and built-in TV, all fully-automated. Many provide video cameras for guests to record their lovemaking and later watch themselves on VCRs. Some rooms are decorated like a wrapped gift or a gigantic windowless egg. Some are conventional—cruise ship cabins or a bed surrounded with stuffed animals. S&M dungeons are the most popular at many, equipped with whips, chains, and cute cartoon characters—the "Kitty S&M Room" features a Kitty-*chan* plush doll wearing a ball gag, blindfold, and barbed wire garter belt. A popular hotel in Osaka has a room with fluorescent wall paintings that appear when the lights are dimmed, making it look like the sea floor or outer space. Psychosexual fantasy options are popular—

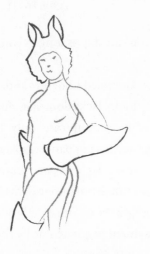

pick the Mercedes-Benz room, teahouse room, hot air balloon room, boxing room, race-car room, or boating room where the boat-bed "floats" in water. An astronaut room comes with space helmets and a space capsule; a jungle room is complete with plastic palm trees, hammock, and a gorilla suit for him. She wears nothing but a smile.

Why not turn *your* bedroom into a love hotel? Hotel sex always seems extra hot. Besides, a quickie can help your relationship. People often have affairs solely for the illicit rush they get from doing something against the rules. Love hotels are places where you can become someone else. Let yourself go and become a Cosplay Girl, "costume play girl"— a hard-core fan of animation, video games, and *manga* comics who dresses up in their latest outfits, such as street-fighting tough chicks, emerald-haired princesses, spunky schoolgirls, and *faux*-fur kittens. Embrace this wacky wannabe subculture with all its glitter, glue, and posing and dress up like your favorite character and invite him to join you in the "party room" of your love hotel.

TURN YOUR BEDROOM INTO A LOVE HOTEL TIPS

- Remove the "homey" atmosphere. Take out office equipment and photos of family and other boyfriends. Paste fluorescent designs onto the ceiling or walls for when the lights go out and the fun begins. Add the touch that every love hotel offers: mirrors overhead, on a Japanese screen, or on your closet doors. Rent some adult videos, and set up your camcorder on a tripod to record the action.

- Buy sheets with the highest threads-per-inch count you can find (two hundred and above). These feel super silky without the cheapness of satin. Decorate your bed with a pillow and sachet. Invest in some thick, fluffy robes or *yukata* (lightweight kimono), and comfy slippers to lounge around in.

- Choose a theme. Love hotels are continuously evolving. Change your motif to go along with your mood *and* your fantasy: an old-fashioned fifties malt shop with a jukebox; a Hollywood film theme with posters, portraits, and videos; a circular bed under a functioning carousel; a traditional *ryokan*, with rice-paper covered sliding doors, *tatami* mats, and a small table with seating cushions; a prison cell; a high school classroom; a UFO; a jungle; a pirate ship; a medieval castle.

- At some love hotels, a computerized concierge greets you with a friendly "Hello, where you been, what's new?" and reminds guests to "come" more often. Greet your lover with your own personal, sexy recorded message.

- Love hotels are redolent of the forbidden. Use scent to set the mood, as well as sound and light features, including a black light. Some hotels have "Body-sonic" in the beds for musical accompaniment and rhythmical help. Pick out your favorite mood music ahead of time and have it cued in at a sexy, but not overpowering, volume.

- A love hotel has an atmosphere of total comfort. Hook up your lighting and sound to easy "on/off" switches. Invest in a small refrigerator filled with favorite treats, a bedroom television with DVD and video, and a hot plate to warm up snacks. Find out what "techno toy" he's pining for to surprise him with when his other toy winds down.

- Guests must take off their shoes before entering the rooms. Have your lover leave his shoes—along with his cell phone and pager—outside the bedroom door.

- If you want a love hotel "Japanese style," buy an inexpensive karaoke machine stocked with favorite sing-alongs.

- Love hotel rooms always have a sex toy vending machine with such "goodies" as dildos, vibrators, and handcuffs. Set up your own display, then let him choose.

- Make a soapland paradise. A bath and shower designed to resemble a mountain stream is very popular, as are dry/steam saunas, Jacuzzi, and rock baths. An excellent selection of makeup, sensual toiletries, and accessories is expected. Install portable fountains in your bathroom for a similar effect, and stock your bathroom with a toothbrush, shaving foam, razors, deodorant, etc. for you and your lover.

- Some love hotels serve soft ice cream cones to every guest and, if you stay the night, a free breakfast. Make a great breakfast (after *you!*) the next morning.

- Many hotels give out Kitty bedside clocks or cute pajamas as souvenirs. Give your man a fun gift before he leaves, like the bottom half of a pair of silk pajamas. He'll be back to see you wearing the top.

Join the fun and put on your black leather outfit. It's up to you if you want to indulge in candle wax dripping on your nipples while you're tied-up and hanging from a hook on the ceiling. Your only limit is your imagination. For the ultimate indulgence, prepare a tray of chilled champagne and his favorite finger foods to savor after you make love. Then pop the video that you made into the VCR and enjoy instant replay.

THE FLOATING WORLD MEETS SEX-ETC.

Sooner the moist and warm leather
Of a good *harigata*,
Than the penis of a blunderer.

Geisha song[36]

While the geisha sought the solitary pleasure of her *harigata* on a hot night under the blue-green mosquito net, the samurai sniffed the sex of his young page; nearby, the shogun wrestled with his passion for female flesh as pink as the peach blossom while he tried to decide which concubine he would bed that night. Life in Old Edo proceeded at its normal pace.

These scenes all speak to the Japanese idea that you have two coexisting souls. Your spiritual soul is uplifting and fulfills your obligations. Your other soul is earthbound, pleasure seeking, and down and dirty. The sensual Japanese woman did not believe the pleasures of the flesh were evil. On the contrary, she believed it was her *right* to enjoy sex in its many different forms. And so should you.

Initiate a sexual move that's both intimate and incredibly sexy and belongs to the two of you alone. It can be both fun and naughty, especially if it's a secret desire you both share. If you want to revitalize the sexual energy of your relationship, moisten your lips and wiggle your hips, because it's time for sex-etc. You will explore everything from sex with more than one partner to homosexuality to auto-erotica to fetishes. Not sure about joining in? You don't have to participate unless you want to, or you can enjoy all the action from the sidelines peeping through your own private spy hole. Let the fun begin.

EROTIC GROUP INTERLUDES

In the late nineteenth century, before a man picked out a girl in a Yoshiwara brothel, he was shown *shashin mitatecho*, a photo album of available prostitutes.[37] More than likely, a man with money to spend picked out several girls to enjoy. Never tried sex with numerous partners? Want to? It's your decision. If you have group sex, you could be inviting the inclusion of partners of a different sexual persuasion. Is this something you have been thinking about? Has he? Not sure? Homosexuality and bisexuality have a long history among the geisha, nuns, and the samurai. Here are some points to consider in deciding if three is your favorite number.

Erotic Group Interludes Tips

- A man who wanted to meet a *tayu* had to go through an intermediary at an expensive tea house. In modern Japan, young women use cell-phone dating sites to find a cybersweetie. You can find modern matchmakers and dating services that specialize in helping *you* find the man or men of your dreams. After meeting with a counselor, you fill out a comprehensive personal profile then tape a short video. When two people show interest in each other after viewing the videos, a meeting is set up.

- For a nominal fee, you can eliminate the intermediary by making an Internet love connection at websites promoting a multi-partner lifestyle. Whether you entertain more than one man in your bed at the same time is up to you.

- The aloof, expensive *tayu* could refuse a client not to her liking. She could break off a relationship if she chose. She might have a special lover for whom she cared deeply. You also have the freedom to choose another if your current bedmate is not to your liking, no matter how many men you have previously taken as lovers, and you are free to have as many bedmates as you like.

- During the Edo period, multiple partners were commonplace among the locals of the countryside during festivals as well as in brothels.[38] A woman might share her man with another female, usually a prostitute. Or, a man might share his wife with other men. If you want to have sex with your man and another woman, you may prefer that she be a professional (in a state or country where this is legal) to avoid him developing any emotional ties with her.

- A popular orgy scene in Old Edo was of a man sodomizing a young man having intercourse with a woman.[39] Choose your partners wisely if you decide to have sex with more than one man at a time. Unless you are willing to participate in bisexual or homosexual liaisons, limit group encounters to those who play the game your way.

- Threesomes were common in the floating world, but one man with two women was more rare than two men sharing a woman.[40] Although your fantasy may be to have two men at the same time, you may find it ego deflating if the men are more interested in each other than they are in you. Lay down the rules ahead of time so you're not disappointed.

- *Shunga* sometimes depict trios with a man having intercourse with a woman as another man takes him from behind. Anal intercourse, known as the "rooster" position,[41] was considered an acceptable pleasure, no matter who was receiving the joy of the man's penis. You may also wish to feel penetration in a dual capacity. Be careful in such situations. Two penises means two condoms. No sharing.

- With group sex, a whole new set of problems and considerations arise if you want to be safe and enjoy yourself at the same time. Don't make the decision lightly. Know all the players in the game, no surprises, and don't exchange body fluids. Ever.

HOMOSEXUAL ENCOUNTERS

Homosexuality was not a punishable offense in Japan until Meiji times. How could it be when it was said that the god "Monju may understand the love of men for men, but he knows little about the love of women."[42] Sodomy was considered a pleasure for men and women, if it was to their taste.

"The Samurai and the *bonze* each know the ways of pleasure; it sometimes happens that they are on it then together."[43] Proud samurai, the professional soldiers who dominated society, revered manly virtues, tough virility, and close-knit comradeship. Dashing and promiscuous even when married, they swore no oath of sexual fidelity and viewed affection for women as a dishonorable sentiment. Passion between males was encouraged. Intercourse between men even had a special term, *ikketsu*.[44] If fallen into the decadent ways of city life, they were as likely to be found at the Kabuki theater where male actors offered their sexual services, as with women in the pleasure quarters. Shaven-headed Buddhist monks were notoriously lecherous. The term *ukiyo bozu* designated a monk who, tired of monastic life, dedicated himself to seeking pleasure. For many, celibacy meant having sexual intercourse not with women, but with young boys.

In the teahouses of Old Edo, a young man's favors could be bought openly. *Wakashu* were boys between the ages of fourteen and seventeen who, having not yet reached manhood, shaved the front part of their head as required by law. Desired by both samurai and monks because their *komon*, anus, was still hairless, they were known as "bamboo shoots" because "they were most tasty when young."[45] The powder-white lubricant *nerigi* was popular with homosexuals, who moistened it with saliva before anal intercourse.

Much about this life went on behind closed shoji. In aristocratic homes, men and women had separate quarters and lived by strict rules. Ladies of the inner apartments seldom saw a man, much less had the opportunity for a love affair. Instead, their needs were serviced by pages, dressed as girls, who performed domestic duties, tea serving, and flower arranging. It has been suggested that these young boys were commanded to have sexual intercourse with the men of the household as well as the women.[46]

Women also engaged in their own games of sexual favors. Homosexuality flourished in the harems of samurai, where sexual frustration and competition ran high. It was also common among the middle classes and in teahouses, where geisha were known to dally with each other. These lesbian relationships were described with the slang term *kai awase*, "the mixing of shellfish."[47] In Ihara Saikaku's novel *Violets Can Be Picked Without Any Trouble,* a famous courtesan, Kosen, thrived on chance encounters with Buddhist nuns.[48] Nuns, in white kimono and with shaved heads, enjoyed fierce love affairs and were widely reputed to turn to prostitution to afford luxuries. This gave rise to the phenomenon of the *ukiyo bikuni*, a prostitute who posed as a nun in order to pursue *her* occupation.[49]

Today, lesbians in Japan are labeled as one of two types: *otachi*, who take on the male role, and *neko*, "cat," or *nenne*, "ingenue."[50] Which role interests you? Not sure? If you are considering a homosexual affair, here are some tips to guide you.

HOMOSEXUAL ENCOUNTERS TIPS

- Like geisha, modern bar hostesses find affairs with women a welcome change from the men they go out with all the time. Women are more gentle and appreciative. If you're tired of how men are treating you or are more aroused by the caresses of a woman, a same-sex relationship may be more fulfilling.

- Geisha endured long separations from their *danna*, protectors, and entered same-sex relationships with little or no guilt. If you're separated from your man for a long period of time and are sexually frustrated, a lighthearted affair with a female friend might be the answer to your needs if your relationships are open.

- Male interest in "girls with girls" was well understood in the floating world and encouraged.[51] Some men find it exciting and stimulating. If you want him to watch you with another girl but don't know how to approach him, try surprising him with a video or reading material depicting your fantasy, then watch his reaction.

- During the Meiji period, to win the approval of the West, homosexuality was made illegal. Whether you decide to engage in a brief homosexual encounter or whether it is a normal part of your life, be aware that a segment of society frowns upon such behavior. Use discretion to protect yourself as well as your lover. Check your local laws.

- In the teahouse, monastery, or harem, a man or a woman did not "become" a homosexual, as the phrase is understood in the West. One encounter does not necessarily make you a lesbian.

Making love with your heart's desire is one of your most profound urges, whichever gender. What about sensual, and often not so subtle, urges and unusual desires that are a bit, well, strange? When is a fetish a fetish? When is it something else?

FETISHES

When a Portuguese ship ran aground on the island of Tanegashima in 1543, the sailors introduced not only firearms but also the word "fetish" into a Japan that looked magical from their perspective. With roots in the Portuguese *feitico* meaning magical practice, and the Latin *factilius*, denoting artificiality, the term was derogatory.[52] No wonder the Portuguese applied it to *shunga*. The exaggerated genitalia of men and women enjoying sexual intercourse were not just exotic to the Portuguese, but artificial-looking. The Japanese did not understand their logic, or lack of it.

According to experts, a fetish is an object or body part that you must focus on to become passionately aroused and, in extreme cases, to achieve orgasm and sexual satisfaction. A fetish can be anything from the well-known fascination for stockings or feet, to "plushophilia," a sexual attraction to furry stuffed toys. The term has evolved from its original meaning to include certain behaviors that can be arousing, such as spanking—whether receiving the sexy slap on the derrière or wielding the whip—or bondage such as *shibari*. Lack of a unity of minds is not uncommon when a fetish is introduced into any relationship. Here are some ideas to help you, odds and ends if you will, about fetishes.

FETISH TIPS

- Black and glossy, a Heian lady's hair tumbled down her back to the floor and, it was said, could snare a man's heart forever. In modern Japan, *kinpatsu*, blonde women, are fetishes. If your man has a fetish about hair, have him give you a scalp massage, rubbing each pressure point in circular motions. *You'll* enter an almost hypnotic state of pleasure, and *he'll* be ready and willing to do just about anything.

- Some Japanese women have a fetish about fishnet tights, using them as a pleasure-seeking sexual tool in which to masturbate to orgasm.

- According to experts, far more men than women have fetishes. In Japan, *chikan*, "gropers," are so common on subways that sex clubs feature mock subway cars complete with hanging straps, taped train noise, and girls who can be pawed for a fee.

- In *shunga*, pubic hair, *chimo*, was drawn in abundance to entice the male eye. The practice was banned in the Meiji period, when Japan imposed a Victorian morality to promote its attempts to catch up with the West.[53] Now, photographs of nude women in men's magazines include it, feeding male obsession over women's genitals. Show him yours, if this is his fetish.

- Many Westerners believe the *unaji*, nape of the geisha's neck, was a fetish. It was not, although geisha pulled their collars down lower than other women. Although many men find backless dresses very sexy, the back is usually not a fetish.

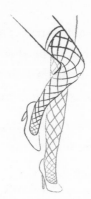

Among some women, fishnet tights are strongly associated with autoeroticism

- The latest sex trend (it could also be considered a fetish for some Japanese men) in Tokyo is *enjo kosai*, meaning "coming to the aid of a young woman by paying for her expenses," that is, compensated dating.[54]

- An extreme fetishist replaces his sexual partner with an object, animate or inanimate, such as a life-size doll. Unless this excites you as well, you'll know your relationship is in trouble if he insists you use a dildo or vibrator more often than his real thing.

- Bondage and fetish go together like whip in hand. In Japanese "mistress bars," the sexy goddess persona of a mistress, dressed in classic latex and leather, dominates men as well as women.

- Photographs of nudes have become so popular since the U.S. Occupation,[55] that some experts now label them a fetish. For a nominal fee at a special studio, a man is supplied with a Polaroid camera, lights, and one or two models. Use a digital camera with your man, but if he spends more time looking at you naked on his computer screen than in bed, cut off his computer connection. *And* him.

• At *nyotai sushi* restaurants, fetishists eat meals served on nude women—giving new meaning to the word "relish."

HENTAI: EROTIC ART COMIX

You'll know that comics are not just for kids if you or your partner is a fan of *hentai*, the wildly popular genre of triple-X cartoons that explore the sexual frontier in an incongru-

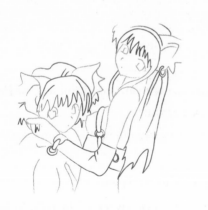

Characters in hentai anime and manga are often exaggerated sexual fantasy figures

ously childlike format. *Hentai* ("perversion") material exploits loopholes in Japanese obscenity laws. Purveyors using words like hard-core, uncut, and uncensored produce films, artwork, digital games, *manga* (comic books), and *anime* (animated films) featuring iconic female characters doing "things unimaginable that will make you explode."[56]

A 1918 code specified the adult "pubic area need not be hidden, but there should be no anatomical details to draw the reader's attention."[57] Instead of blocking pornography, it inspired illustrators to thwart the law by depicting sexual organs in shadow or outline, colored blue or green—signifying they could not possibly be human—or, as part of a monster. In recent years, animators have drawn female characters that look like preteens. Devoid of pubic hair, they theoretically are outside the boundaries of the regulation. Childlike to Western eyes, to Japanese males the distinction is not as clear.

The ultimate fantasy of Japanese males is the *jogakusei*, a virginal schoolgirl. Over time, the seduction or sexual transgression of girlish characters has evolved into a socially acceptable, modern version of the Old Edo floating world *shunga*. The star of a *hentai* film or *manga* is typically a perky, doe-eyed female in a high school uniform. Her exploits are a mix of graphic violence and weird sex, drawn explicitly. The costars of the big-breasted, pink-skinned *hentai* heroines range from slobbering businessmen and sado-masochistic school officials to hormonal extraterrestrials. With its oversexed and bigger-than-life drawings, *hentai* has a worldwide following. Introduce your man to the heroines of *hentai* and he'll think he's a teenager again. Hopefully, he will act like one where it counts.

A FLOWER BLOSSOMS . . .

Close your eyes and let your thoughts wander. Take a deep, cleansing breath. Feels good. You have discovered the secrets to the art of seduction and made them your own. Yet, your path to enlightenment is not over. As the fourteenth-century author Urabe Kenko wrote in *Idle Hours*, "Pleasure . . . loving someone and becoming attached to someone; an endless quest."[1]

What does this mean? Simply that every love affair is different, and requires all the skills you have learned in this book to make it sensual and extraordinary. Think of yourself as a geisha who has studied the art of dance for years with her *sensei*. She learns every pattern, every technique, but when she goes out on stage, unfolds her fan, and begins to dance, she is on her own.

You have studied geisha, courtesans, and Heian ladies and learned their secrets in the art of seduction, but the dance you perform is yours alone.

Dance it well.

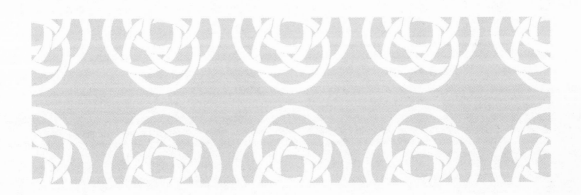

NOTES

For each chapter, notes for sidebars are lettered and follow the numbered notes for the main text.

INTRODUCTION

1. Ruth Benedict, *The Chrysanthemum and the Sword* (Japan: Charles Tuttle, 1954), 283.

JAPANESE WOMEN THROUGHOUT THE AGES

1. Joan Mellen, *The Waves at Genji's Door* (New York: Pantheon Books, 1976), 12, 392.
2. Ryusaku Tsunoda, Wm. Theodore de Bary, and Donald Keene, *Sources of Japanese Tradition*, Volume I (New York: Columbia University Press, 1964), 42.
3. Eliza Ruhamah Scidmore, *Jinrikisha Days in Japan* (New York, London: Harper and Brothers, 1891), 310.
4. Sara M. Harvey, "The Juni-hito of Heian Japan," http://www.clotheslinejournal.com/heian.html.
5. Donald Keene, *Anthology of Japanese Literature* (New York: Grove Press, 1955), 156.
6. Bernard Soulié, *Japanese Erotism* (New York: Crescent Books, 1981), 8.
7. Earl Roy Miner, Robert E. Morrell, and Hiroko Odagiri, *The Princeton Companion to Classical Japanese Literature* (Princeton: Princeton Univer-

sity Press, 1988), 289.
8. Tsunoda, et al., *Sources of Japanese Tradition*, Volume I, 174.
9. Eleanor Underwood, *The Life of a Geisha* (New York: Smithmark, 1999), 15.
10. Tom and Mary Anne Evans, *Shunga: The Art of Love,* reprint (New York: Paddington Press, 1975), 30.
11. Ihara Saikaku, *Life of an Amorous Woman*, edited and translated by Ivan Morris (New York: New Directions, Unesco, 1963), 295.
12. Nicholas Bornoff, *Pink Samurai* (New York: Pocket Books, 1991), 239–40.
13. Lesley Downer, *Women of the Pleasure Quarters* (New York: Broadway Books, 2001), 99.
14. "Japan: Wireless for Sex," Tech TV: Wired for Sex, http://www.techtv.com/wiredforsex/shownotes/story/0,24330,3446243,00.html.

a. Tsunoda, et al., *Sources of Japanese Tradition*, Volume I, 43.
b. Evans, *Shunga*, 27.
c. Tsunoda, et al., *Sources of Japanese Tradition*, Volume I, 435.

CHAPTER ONE: KOKONO-TOKORO, "THE NINE POINTS OF BEAUTY"

1. Howard A. Link, *Japanese Genre Paintings from*

the Kyusei Atami Art Museum (Tokyo: Benrido, 1980–81), 26.

2. Saikaku, *Life of an Amorous Woman*, 355.

3. Jorgen Andersen-Rosendal, *The Moon of Beauty* (New York: John Day, 1957), 13–14.

4. Link, *Japanese Genre Paintings*, 25.

5. As related by Dr. Caron Smith, SDMA Curator of European Art, San Diego Museum of Art, San Diego, California, July 12, 2001.

6. Kikou Yamata, *Three Geishas* (New York: John Day, 1956), 104.

7. Kyoko Aihara, *World of the Geisha* (Dubai: Carlton Books, 1999), 77.

8. Saikaku, *Life of an Amorous Woman*, 303.

9. Ibid., 354.

10. Keene, *Anthology of Japanese Literature*, 335.

11. Downer, *Women of the Pleasure Quarters*, 6, 47.

12. Aihara, *World of the Geisha*, 77.

13. Saikaku, *Life of an Amorous Woman*, 132.

14. Michelle D. Leigh, *The Japanese Way of Beauty: Natural Beauty and Health Secrets* (New York: Carol Publishing Group, 1992), 13.

15. Hisayo Grace Maeda and Lucille Craft, *Japanese Secrets of Beautiful Skin and Weight Control: The Maeda Program* (Boston: Tuttle Publishing, 1995), 194.

16. Leigh, *Japanese Way of Beauty*, 15–16.

17. Keene, *Anthology of Japanese Literature*, 149.

18. Leigh, *Japanese Way of Beauty*, 88.

19. Cecilia Segawa Seigle, *Yoshiwara: The Glittering World of the Japanese Courtesan* (Honolulu: Uni-versity of Hawaii Press, 1993), 192.

20. Downer, *Women of the Pleasure Quarters*, 114.

21. Liza Crihfield Dalby, *Geisha* (Berkeley: University of California Press, 1983), 45–46.

22. Leigh, *Japanese Way of Beauty*, 99.

23. Hendrik De Leeuw, *Cities of Sin* (New York: Wil-ley Book Company, 1933), 37.

24. Seigle, *Yoshiwara*, 77.

25. Saikaku, *Life of an Amorous Woman*, 132.

26. Leigh, *Japanese Way of Beauty*, 191.

27. Downer, *Women of the Pleasure Quarters*, 108.

28. Maeda, *Japanese Secrets of Beautiful Skin and Weight Control*, 196–98.

29. Michel Beurdeley, *Erotic Art* (Hong Kong: Leon Amiel Publisher, n.d.), 145–46.

30. De Leeuw, *Cities of Sin,* 61.

31. Ibid., 32.

32. Downer, *Women of the Pleasure Quarters*, 239.

33. Link, *Japanese Genre Paintings*, 39.

34. Evans, *Shunga*, 284.

35. Saikaku, *Life of an Amorous Woman*, 339.

36. Beurdeley, *Erotic Art*, 145–46.

37. Link, *Japanese Genre Paintings*, 14.

38. Andersen-Rosendal, *Moon of Beauty*, 105.

39. Fosco Maraini, *Meeting with Japan* (New York: Viking Press, 1960), 347.

40. Mrs. Hugh Fraser, *The Heart of a Geisha* (New York: Putnam, 1908), 69.

41. De Leeuw, *Cities of Sin*, 35.

42. Andersen-Rosendal, *Moon of Beauty*, 105.

43. Robert Lyons Daly, *In the Shade of Spring Leaves* (New Haven, London: Yale University Press, 1975), 94.

a. Downer, *Women of the Pleasure Quarters*, 87.

b. Dalby, *Geisha*, 133.

c. Anonymous, *Geisha Secrets: A Pillow Book for Lovers* (New York: Carroll and Graf, 2000), 15.

d. Downer, *Women of the Pleasure Quarters*, 85.

e. Aihara, *World of the Geisha*, 77.

f. Anonymous, *Geisha Secrets*, 15.

g. Downer, *Women of the Pleasure Quarters*, 86, 239.

h. Daily Candy LA, Drinks and Food, www.Dailycandy.com, May 18, 2002.

i. Saikaku, *Life of an Amorous Woman*, 307.

j. Ibid., 318.

k. Dalby, *Geisha*, 86.

l. Downer, *Women of the Pleasure Quarters*, 6.

m. Ibid., 187.

n. Aihara, *World of the Geisha*, 40.

o. Scidmore, *Jinrikisha Days in Japan*, 214–15.

p. Fraser, *Heart of a Geisha*, 25.

q. Christine Arnothy, *Women of Japan* (London: André Deutsch, 1959), 26.

CHAPTER TWO: BATHING PLEASURES

1. Maeda, *Japanese Secrets of Beautiful Skin and Weight Control*, 111.

2. Ibid., 112.

3. Richard Boeke, Rev. Yopie Boeke, Yuji Inokuma, "An American Religionist Experiences Shinto," http://www.csuchico.edu/~georgew/tsa/nl/f95p2.html.

4. Mildred Watt, *Japan, Land of Sun and Storm* (Boston, Toronto: Ginn and Company, 1966), 187.

5. Beurdeley, *Erotic Art*, 264.

6. Soulié, *Japanese Erotism*, 69.

7. Jordan Sand, editor, *Yanesen Magazine*, no. 1 (Tokyo: Sanseisha), p. 2.

8. Maeda, *Japanese Secrets of Beautiful Skin and Weight Control*, 112.

9. Lewis Bush, *Bathhouse Nights* (Japan: Tokyo News Service, 1958), 3.

10. Ibid., 7.

11. Jack Seward, *The Japanese* (Lincolnwood, Illinois: Passport Books, 1971), 47.

a. Leigh, *Japanese Way of Beauty*, 146.

b. Ibid., 131.

c. Ibid., 139.

CHAPTER THREE: EROTIC MEDITATION

1. http://www.geocities.com/Paris/5870/ikk.html.

2. Dr. Elizabeth A. Weidlich, "Manage Stress with Proper Breathing," *Los Alamitos Sun*, October 4, 2001, 15.

3. Beurdeley, *Erotic Art*, 263.

4. F. Hadland Davis, *Myths and Legends of Japan* (New York: Dover Publications, 1992), 293.

5. Paul Varley and Kumakura Isao, editors, *Tea in Japan: Essays on the History of Chanoyu* (Honolulu: University of Hawaii Press, 1989), 5.

6. Oliver Statler, *All-Japan: The Catalogue of Every-*

thing Japanese (New York: Quarto Marketing, 1984), 96.

a. Dalby, *Geisha*, 90.

b. Passler's Top-Shape Tips, *Harper's Bazaar* (New York: September 2002), 186.

CHAPTER FOUR: INTOXICATING MOOD ENHANCERS

1. Beurdeley, *Erotic Art*, 70.

2. Patricia Davis, "New Look, Same Old Stuff: House-Fluffing Is the Rage with Budget-Minded Clients Demand for $300 Quick-Fix," *Wall Street Journal*, November 15, 2002, B1.

3. Scidmore, *Jinrikisha Days in Japan*, 280.

4. Dalby, *Geisha*, 331.

5. Ibid., 327.

6. Beurdeley, *Erotic Art*, 40.

7. Author unknown, *Famous Women: Comparative Portraits of Their Devotion* (1681), quoted in Beurdeley, *Erotic Art*, 106.

8. Scidmore, *Jinrikisha Days in Japan*, 274.

9. Chris Knap, "Uncorked: Warm up to Fine Sake—Now Chilled."*Orange County Register*, February 6, 2000, Food 1.

10. *Natural History*, August 1993, 60.

11. John David Morley, *Pictures from the Water Trade* (New York: Harper and Row, 1985), 256.

CHAPTER FIVE: IKI, THE ART OF COOL

1. Quoted in Underwood, *Life of a Geisha*, 11. Originally appeared in Liza Crihfield, *Ko-uta:*

Little Songs of the Geisha World (Tokyo: Charles E. Tuttle, 1979), 67.

2. Dalby, *Geisha*, 272.

3. Ibid., 273.

4. Kittredge Cherry, *Womansword: What Japanese Words Say About Women* (Tokyo: Kodansha International, 1987), 25.

5. Saikaku, *Life of an Amorous Woman*, 138.

6. Beurdeley, *Erotic Art*, 145.

7. Anonymous, *Geisha Secrets*, 45.

8. Kyoto Fusuishi, *The Smiling Faces of Pleasure Seekers* (1778), quoted in Beurdeley, *Erotic Art*, 216.

9. *Discover Japan, Volume 1: Words, Customs, and Concepts* (New York and San Francisco: Kodansha International, 1982), 102.

10. Pierre Landy, *The Japan I Love*, translated from the French by Ruth Whipple Fermaud (New York: Tudor, 1965), 10.

11. Quoted in Beurdeley, *Erotic Art*, 134.

a. *Shotesu Monogatari,* in *Zoku Gunsho Ruiju*, Book 13, 929 quoted in Tsunoda, et al., *Sources of Japanese Tradition*, Volume I, 279.

CHAPTER SIX: THE ART OF PLAY

1. Underwood, *Life of a Geisha*, 48. Originally appeared in R. H. Blyth, *Edo Satirical Verse Anthologies* (Tokyo: Hokuseido Press, 1961), 17.

2. Fraser, *Heart of a Geisha*, 17.

3. Saikaku, *Life of an Amorous Woman*, 339.

4. Yamata, *Three Geishas*, 129.

5. Beurdeley, *Erotic Art,* 177.

6. Mark Magnier, "Compliments Available for a Price on Tokyo Streets, *Los Angeles Times,* Southern California Living, May 23, 2000, E1.

7. Theresa O'Rourke, "Lust Lessons," *Cosmopolitan,* January 2003, 86.

8. Benedict, *Chrysanthemum and the Sword,* 186.

9. Sand,*Yanesen Magazine,* no. 1, 2.

10. Boye Lafayette De Mente, *Japan Made Easy,* 2nd edition (Lincolnwood, Illinois: Passport Books, 1995), 127.

11. Ibid., 123.

12. Bornoff, *Pink Samurai,* 270.

13. http://www.taidemuseo.hel.fi/suomi/tennispalatsi/lisat/2shungaenglpuup.html.

14. Bornoff, *Pink Samurai,* 135.

15. Beurdeley, *Erotic Art,* 144.

16. Ibid., 262.

17. Deborah Sundahl, *Female Ejaculation and The G-SPOT (*Alameda, California: Hunter House, 2003), 57.

18. Evans, *Shunga,* 45.

19. Joseph Coleman, "Japanese City Caters to Daring Fugu Lovers," *Orange County Register,* December 31, 2000, News 30.

20. Japan Culture Institute, *Discover Japan,* 198.

a. Japan America Friendship Foundation and U.S.-Japan Network, *Japan: Then and Now,* November 1992, 77.

b. Romance Writers of America, Orange County Meeting, December 14, 2002.

c. Nicole Beland, "Create Your Own Red-Light District, " *Cosmopolitan,* Luxe-life Tip, June 2002, 138.

CHAPTER SEVEN: SEEDING THE FLOWER AND TWIRLING THE STEM

1. Beurdeley, *Erotic Art,* 204.

2. Soulié, *Japanese Erotism,* 6.

3. Ed Jacob, "Japan's Quirky Festivals," *Japanzine,* March 2003), http://www3.tky.3web.ne.jp/~edjacob/index.html.

4. Evans, *Shunga,* 46.

5. Ibid., 78.

6. Beurdeley, *Erotic Art,* 261.

7. William Fitzpatrick, *Tokyo After Dark* (New York: Macfadden-Bartell Corporation, 1965), 16.

8. Beurdeley, *Erotic Art,* 261.

9. Ibid., 200.

10. Underwood, *Life of a Geisha,* 9–10.

11. Dalby, *Geisha,* 109.

12. Ibid., 109.

13. Underwood, *Life of a Geisha,* 42.

14. Beurdeley, *Erotic Art,* 261–63.

15. Ibid., 180–81.

16. Bornoff, *Pink Samurai,* 75.

17. Anonymous, *Geisha Secrets,* 36.

18. Quoted in Daly, *In the Shade of Spring Leaves,* 162.

19. Beurdeley, *Erotic Art,* 173.

20. Saikaku, *Life of an Amorous Woman,* 332, n. 317.

21. Beurdeley, *Erotic Art,* 231.

22. Mia, "Sex in the World of the Japanese Mind: Guide to Sex with a Japanese Man," http://www.mynippon.com/romance/sex_guide.htm.

23. Ibid.

24. Anonymous, *Geisha Secrets,* 36.

25. Cherry, *Womansword,* 117.

26. Anonymous, *Geisha Secrets,* 44.

27. Anonymous, *Fukujuso, Sixteen Erotic Tales,* 1778, quoted in Beurdeley, *Erotic Art,* 212.

28. Soulié, *Japanese Erotism,* 94.

29. Cherry, *Womansword,* 36.

30. Anonymous, *Geisha Secrets,* 36.

31. *The Alternative Japanese Dictionary,* http://www.notam.uio.no/~hcholm/altlang/ht/Japanese.html.

32. Sundahl, *Female Ejaculation and The G-SPOT,* 57.

33. Beurdeley, *Erotic Art,* 200.

34. Ibid., 180.

35. Ibid., 252.

36. Anonymous, *Geisha Secrets,* 40.

37. Cherry, *Womansword,* 33.

38. Soulié, *Japanese Erotism,* 78–79.

a. Evans, *Shunga,* 51.

b. Beurdeley, *Erotic Art,* 131.

c. Anonymous, *Geisha Secrets,* 36.

d. Valentin Chu, *The Yin-Yang Butterfly* (New York: G. P. Putnam's Sons, 1993), 109–13.

CHAPTER EIGHT: NAKED GAMES

1. Bornoff, *Pink Samurai,* 316.

2. Ibid., 310.

3. Evans, *Shunga,* 30.

4. Ibid., 52.

5. Bornoff, *Pink Samurai,* 310.

6. Evans, *Shunga,* 52.

7. Mark Magnier, "The World: Blaze Kills 44 in Tokyo Adult District," *Los Angeles Times,* September 1, 2001, A1.

8. Bornoff, *Pink Samurai,* 313.

9. Ibid., 31.

10. Soulié, *Japanese Erotism,* 21.

11. Christopher C. McGooey, "Shogun Sex," *Penthouse Forum* (New York: Forum International), April 1987, 29.

12. Dalby, *Geisha,* 55.

13. "Japanese Bondage," http://en.wikipedia.org/wiki/Shibari.

14. "Shibari: Technique for Kinky Sex in Japan," http://www.mynippon.com/romance/shibari.htm.

15. "Terms," http://www.ds-arts.com/RopeArt/Terms.html.

16. Ibid.

17. Beurdeley, *Erotic Art,* 195.

18. Evans, *Shunga,* 51.

19. Anonymous, *Geisha Secrets,* 31.

20. Masquerade Erotic Newsletter, "Sexual Freedom in Japan," July/August 1993.

21. "Terms," http://www.ds-arts.com/RopeArt/

Terms.html.

22. Bornoff, *Pink Samurai*, 158.

23. Ibid., 438.

24. Magnier, "Blaze Kills 44," A1.

25. Bornoff, *Pink Samurai*, 273.

26. Ibid., 159.

27. Author unknown, *Famous Women: Comparative Portraits of Their Devotion,* 1681, quoted in Beurdeley, *Erotic Art,* 262.

28. Bornoff, *Pink Samurai*, 158.

29. Alex Comfort, M.D., *The Joy of Sex* (New York: Crown, 1991), 156.

30. Evans, *Shunga*, 52.

31. Beurdeley, *Erotic Art,* 263.

32. "Life-Size Tokimeki Memorial 2 Dolls," http://ps2.ign.com/articles/101/101266p1.html?fromint=1.

33. "A Beginner's Guide To The Japanese Zodiac," Japan Visitor, http://japanvisitor.com/jc/zodiac.html.

34. Real Doll, http://www.realdoll.com/faq.asp (prices as of 2003).

35. Andreas Stuhlmann, "Between a Rock and a Soft Place," Tokyo Journal, http://www.tokyo.to/backissues/apr00/tj0400p6-10/index.html.

36. Soulié, *Japanese Erotism*, 81.

37. Emmett Murphy, *Great Bordellos of the World* (London: Quartet Books, 1983), 149.

38. Bornoff, *Pink Samurai*, 186.

39. Evans, *Shunga*, 49.

40. Bornoff, *Pink Samurai*, 186–87.

41. Woodblock Print Series 8: Isoda Koryusai, "Glories of the Twelve Months (Furyu juni-ki no eiga)," set of 12, chuban, 1773, http://www.taidemuseo.hel.fi/english/tennispalatsi/programme/shunga.html.

42. Keene, *Anthology of Japanese Literature*, 350.

43. Soulié, *Japanese Erotism*, 57.

44. Beurdeley, *Erotic Art*, 262.

45. Evans, *Shunga*, 49.

46. James Cleugh, *Oriental Orgies: An Account of Some Erotic Practices Among Non-Christians* (London: Anthony Blond, 1968), 188.

47. Bornoff, *Pink Samurai*, 438.

48. Beurdeley, *Erotic Art*, 163.

49. Ibid., 263.

50. Bornoff, *Pink Samurai*, 438.

51. Anonymous, *Geisha Secrets*, 31.

52. David Pagel, "Once-Powerful Fetishes Open the Door to Their World: In 'Fetish: Art/Word,' Contemporary Works Are Juxtaposed with African Artifacts in a Look at the Power of Symbols and the History of the Word," *Los Angeles Times,* Art Review, June 22, 2002, Calendar F18.

53. Merrill Goozner, "Sex in Japan Is Flourishing—But It's Kept under Wraps," *Orange County Register,* June 18, 1995, News 24.

54. "Japan: Wireless for Sex," Tech TV: Wired for Sex.

55. Maraini, *Meeting with Japan*, 59.

56. http://www.hentaipop.com/preview/ January 2003.

57. P. J. Huffstutter, "X-Rated Fantasies in a Cartoon

Genre; Japan's Hentai Films, with Doe-eyed Characters and Bizarre Sexuality, Find a U.S. Market," *Los Angeles Times,* Southern California Living, June 13, 2002, E1.

AFTERWORD: A FLOWER BLOSSOMS

1. Beurdeley, *Erotic Art,* 71.

GLOSSARY

amado: outside wooden doors

azuki: small, dark red, and oval, delicately flavored beans

bento: box lunch

bobokai: "shell," metaphor for vulva

byobu: folding screen

cha: tea

chado: "The Way of Tea"

chanoyu: tea ceremony

dohan: "couples dates"

enjo kosai: compensated dating

fugu: pufferfish

furin: wind chimes

fusuma: sliding wall panels

geiko: "geisha" in Kyoto dialect

geisha: "arts person," from *gei*, "art," and *sha*, "person"

geisha-ya: geisha teahouse

girichoco: "obligation chocolate" given by women to men on Valentine's Day

hadaka matsuri: "naked" festivals

hana: flower

hanadai: "flower money"; fee paid for the services of a geisha

hanafuda: card game with forty-eight cards, each decorated with a flower design

hanamachi: "flower towns"; geisha sections

hanko: name stamp

haori: a kimono-style jacket worn over a kimono for added warmth

hara: belly

hari: seductive spirit

harigata: dildo

hashi: low-class prostitute

hentai: erotic art comix

hinoki: cypress

honmeichoco: chocolate more expensive than *girichoco*; can be homemade.

horimono: tattoo

horoyoi: slightly intoxicated

hosutesu: bar hostesses

ikebana: flower arranging

iki: erotic sense of style and polish exemplified by certain geisha and courtesans; art of "cool"

irome kasane: art of multi-layering of colors

itoke: sex appeal

jaku: tranquillity

janken-pon: "scissors cut paper, paper wraps stone, stone breaks scissors" game played at geisha banquets

jokyu: cafe girls

kado: flower arranging

kaiseki: elegant multi-course meal

kanji: pictograms of Chinese origin used in modern Japanese

kanzashi: silver hair pins

karakasa: brightly colored and lightweight parasol made from oiled-paper, silk, and bamboo

karyukai: "world of flowers and willows"

kei: respect

ko: incense

kokono-tokoro: nine points of beauty

koro: incense burner

kotatsu: low, quilt-covered table with a heat source below

koto: thirteen-stringed harp

maiko: apprentice geisha

maiogi: fan with bamboo spines about twelve inches long used by a geisha when she danced

Makura no Soshi: Pillow Book

maneki neko: "beckoning cats" statues found in geisha houses

matcha: vivid green powder of ground tea leaves that makes a frothy green tea

matsuke: penis; mushroom

matsuri: festivals

mayu: eyebrows

meishi: business cards

meishoki: guidebooks

misemono: sideshows

miyabi: courtly beauty

mizuage: "drawing from the water"; defloration ceremony of a *maiko*

mizushobai: "water trade"; sex business

mono no aware: deep feeling prompted by the experience of extreme beauty

mu: non-existence

nagajuban: kimono underslip

nerigi: powder-white lubricant produced from sea algae and mallow roots

noren: entry curtains

nuka: rice bran

obi: wide sash worn around the waist and midsection

obijime: cord encircling a geisha's sash

ochoboguchi: small mouth

odoriko: "dancing child"; young female entertainers

ofuku: less decorative *maiko* hairstyle with the knot lower down

ofuro: bath

ogi: folding fan

ohana: "honorable flower"; fee paid for the services of a geisha

oiran: courtesan

okami-san: teahouse owner

okasan: mama-san

okiya: teahouse

okobo: six-inch high clogs with tinkling bells worn by *maiko*

omakase: tasting menu

onesan: older geisha sister

onsen: hot springs resorts

oshiroi: white geisha makeup

ozashiki: geisha banquets

panko: Japanese-style bread crumbs made from bleached wheat flour, soy bean oil, palm oil, yeast, and salt

potchiri: sash clasp

rabu hoteru, rabu-ho: love hotel

rin no tama: benwa balls

rotenburo: outdoor bath located in a scenic spot

ryokan: traditional Japanese-style inn

saburuko: ones who serve

sakeburo: sake bath

sansuke: masseur

sei: purity

seiko: sex
sensei: teacher
sento: community bathhouse
seppun: kiss
shakuhachi: flute
shakuhachi o fuku: "blowing the flute"; oral sex
shamisen: three-stringed lute
shiatsu: finger-pressure massage
shibari: erotic bondage
shijuhachi te: "forty-eight ways"; sexual positions based on the ways a sumo wrestler can defeat his opponent
shikishi: rectangular or fan-shaped writing papers used to mark special occasions.
shinju: lovers' suicide
shoji: translucent paper doors or windows
shunga: "spring drawings"; erotic art of the Edo period
sudare: reed curtain
sumo: combat between two people who can use nothing but their bodies
sumotori: sumo wrestlers
tabi: white socks worn with *geta*
tatami: straw mat used as flooring in teahouses
tayu: highest-ranking courtesan in Old Edo
tenugui: linen cloth about the size of a small guest towel for both washing and drying
tokonoma: position of honor
toro: tuna
uchigi: outer robe worn over a kimono
uchiwa: flat fans with handles
ukiyo: "the floating world"
ukiyoe: woodblock prints from the Edo period
umami: glutamate-inspired, deliciously savory sensation
wa: harmony
wabi: understated elegance
wakame: seaweed
wareme-chan: "dear little slit"; clitoris
wareshinobu: *maiko* maiden hairstyle, characterized by a bagel-shaped, rolled knot worn high on her head, decorated with ribbons, ornaments, and silk flowers
washi: handmade paper used for writing letters
yakuza: Japanese mafia
yoin: sound a bell makes after it is struck; a resonance
yoisho: art of giving subtle compliments
yugen: quiet beauty; elegant simplicity
yujo: prostitute
yukata: loose-fitting cotton kimono
yuna: bath maiden
yuzu: yellow citron

INDEX

JINA BACARR has written business books and magazine and newspaper articles about Japan. She was the Japanese consultant on KCBS-TV, MSNBC, Tech TV's Wired for Sex, and British Sky Broadcasting Ltd.'s Saucy TV, and has appeared in Japanese commercials, worked as a companion girl for a Japanese company, and studied the art of kimono with a teacher whose family has been in the kimono business for 400 years. She was the Lifestyles Editor on "The Tony Trupiano Show" on Talk America Radio Network, a late-night radio jock, and produced and hosted her own weekly radio show "On the Wild Side," the spicier side of books, on Book Crazy Radio. A graduate of UC Irvine, Jina speaks French, German, Italian, Spanish, and conversational Japanese. She has had three plays produced and has written more than forty scripts for daytime television (including thirty animation scripts). She has also taught a college course about women in Japan. Jina Bacarr's website is at www.SuzyIQ.com.

OTHER STONE BRIDGE PRESS TITLES OF INTEREST

The Japanese Home Stylebook: Architectural Details and Motifs by Saburo Yamagata

Designing with Kanji: Japanese Character Motifs for Surface, Skin & Spirit
by Shogo Oketani and Leza Lowitz

Shinto Meditations for Revering the Earth by Stuart D. B. Picken

Saké Pure + Simple by Griffith Frost and John Gauntner

Living the Japanese Arts & Ways: 45 Paths to Meditation & Beauty by H. E. Davey

Wabi-Sabi: for Artists, Designers, Poets & Philosophers by Leonard Koren

Yoga Poems: Lines to Unfold By by Leza Lowitz

A String of Flowers Untied . . . Love Poems from "The Tale of Genji" by Murasaki Shikibu

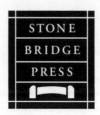

Stone Bridge Press publishes fine books about Japan and Asia.
We welcome your comments and suggestions. Write to us at sbp@stonebridge.com.

STONE BRIDGE PRESS • P. O. BOX 8208 • BERKELEY, CALIFORNIA 94707

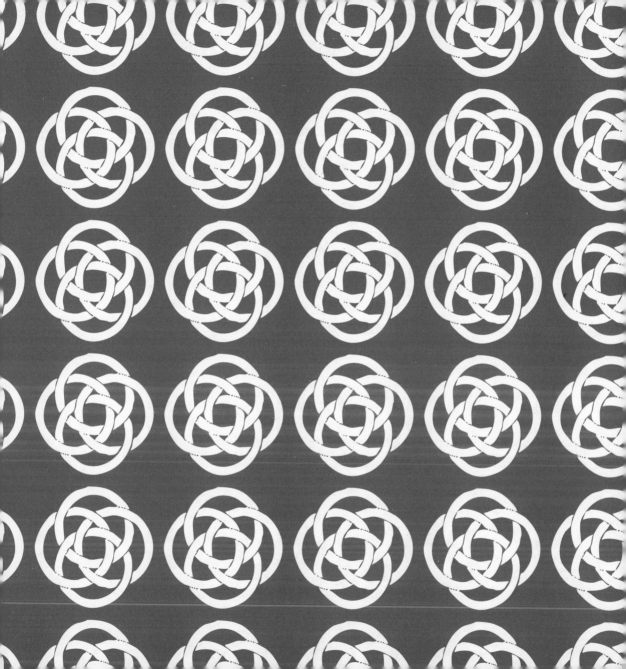

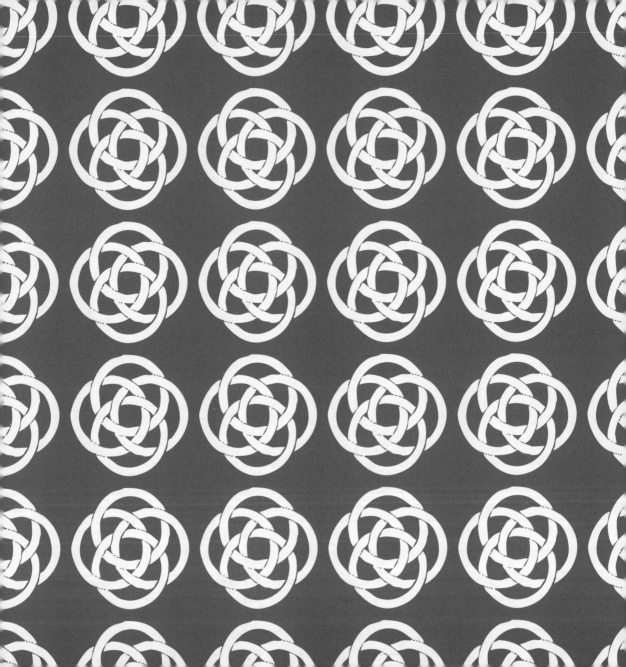